Dun 01/17.

0 8 MAR 2017

1 3 MAY 2

D0716902

The hope of humanity lies in the prevention of degenerative and mental diseases, not in the care of their symptoms.

Dr Alexis Carrel

To All Health Seekers

Also from Carlton
the companion title

COMPLETE NUTRITION
How to Live in Total Health

Dr Michael Sharon

THE COMPLETE GUIDE TO
Nutrients

Dr Michael Sharon

An A–Z of superfoods, herbs, vitamins, minerals and supplements

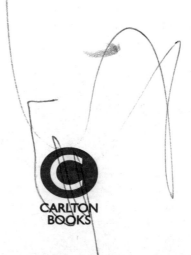

CARLTON
BOOKS

This seventh edition published in 2017
by Carlton Books Limited
20 Mortimer Street
London W1T 3JW

First published in 1998 by Prion Books Ltd

10 9 8 7 6 5 4 3 2 1

A CIP catalogue record for this book is available from the British Library

ISBN 978 1 78097 904 5

Printed and bound in the UK by CPI Group (UK) Ltd, Croydon, CR0 4YY

*This book has been designed as a quick reference dictionary for nutritional information.
Its contents are strictly educative and are not intended to be diagnostic or prescriptive. The
publishers, author and editors do not imply or intend that this book should in any way
replace medical consultation or the services of a physician.*

PREFACE

Nutritional knowledge is in high demand. 'Back to nature' awareness has become a way of life for many thousands of people and nutritional supplements, organic produce, health foods and rediscovered herbs are the talk of the day. People are taking more responsibility for their own well-being and the result is a greater need for nutritional information, conveniently available and easily understood.

This book is intended to serve as a nutritional dictionary, a quick reference book for lay people as well as professionals. It is meant to provide basic information on various nutritional issues, and can easily be used at home or while shopping in the health food store.

We each react differently to foods, and this includes health foods, nutrients and herbs. Sometimes, we even have opposite effects and reactions. This should be remembered when trying a supplement for the first time: nutrients and herbs must be adapted to the individual. It should also be remembered that the information included in this book is based on average effects that apply to most people, but not necessarily to everybody. Most important of all – do not self-diagnose. In cases of conditions suggestive of symptoms discussed in this book, please consult a natural health care specialist or a holistic doctor for professional advice.

Following the success of its more comprehensive predecessor, *Complete Nutrition*, I hope that this new book will serve to increase public awareness of the exciting connection between nutrition, well-being and longevity. Due to misinformation, many people unknowingly consume harmful foods which act as an enemy. Let us make food our ally. In the words of Hippocrates, 'Let us make food our medicine'.

My acknowledgements go to Deborah Ackland MSc, for her continuous advice and support; to my publisher Barry Winkleman, the inspiring force behind this publication; and to my dedicated editors Andrew Goodfellow and Mary Warren, who together spared no effort in editing the manuscript. May they all be blessed.

Dr Michael Sharon

HOW TO SOURCE YOUR NUTRIENTS

The various nutrients outlined in the following pages – fruit, vegetables, oils, herbs, vitamins, minerals and supplements – can be found in a wide variety of locations from the obvious to the less obvious. Increasingly, supermarkets and grocers are stocking a wider variety of produce from around the world and many of the foods, herbs and spices that were once thought of as rare can now be readily located with a minimum of effort. As health becomes more of an issue too, foods with a healing dimension are increasingly available in supermarkets, local stores and grocers.

For more specialist nutrients you may need to take a trip to your local health food store where help and advice is available. Here, in addition to nutritious foods and herbs, you will find a multitude of vitamins, minerals and nutrients in capsule form and the many compound nutritional formulas that are often tailored toward helping a specific condition. Health food stores obviously vary in size and some of the more specialist nutrients may be available only from larger outlets. Pharmacies also increasingly serve the health food market with a wide range of vitamins, minerals and supplements.

Specialist herbs may again be harder to find, especially fresh herbs. Whereas the health food shop is an increasingly familiar sight on our streets and may offer a range of herbal products, the herbalist is still something of a rarity. At the back of the book is a list of helpful addresses which includes herbalist associations that can offer general advice, herbal suppliers and mail-order companies in both the UK and the USA.

Information on sourcing a nutrient is contained within each individual entry. For dosage you should always consult the instructions on the packaging and, for specific conditions, always consult a knowledgeable medical practitioner.

Within the following A to Z, as well as entries on every kind of nutrient, there are also entries on key terms and more general topics within the field of nutrition. They are intended to go some way in helping to guide the reader through the vast field of information available on the subject.

Where relevant, within each entry, some of the other key terms or nutrients discussed have been marked in bold to let the reader know that there is a separate entry in the book on that particular subject.

The index at the back of the book complements the main A to Z by covering all the medical and health complaints that are mentioned within these nutritional entries.

A

ACAI (*EUTERPE OLERACEA*)

Growing in huge clusters on the acai palm tree, acai berries are native to Brazil and were used for centuries by the Amazon tribes. Recently, they became internationally popularized as a superfood. The berries are indeed a storehouse of nutrients, loaded with vitamins, minerals, essential fatty acids and fibre. But more importantly, acai berries have been found to contain ultra high concentrations of polyphenolic antioxidants, including anthocyanin and proanthocyanidins, a group of flavonoid pigments that give the berries their deep purple colour. Studies indicated that their strong antioxidant effects protect body cells from free radicals damage, boost the immune system, support cardiovascular health, and even slow down ageing. (Acai berries are very perishable, which is why they must be freeze-dried within 24 hours to preserve their goodness.)

ACID-ALKALINE BALANCE

Although the body has its own natural acid-alkaline balancing mechanisms, an over-indulgence of acidic foods – especially the rich and spicy foods that tend to form the basis of the modern Western diet – can impair this delicate balance. A healthy body needs to be slightly alkaline (pH 7.35–7.45) to counteract these effects. This alkalinity serves as a natural buffer against acid-forming conditions such as stress, lack of exercise, poor eating habits and chronic constipation.

The digestion of acid-forming foods (**meat, fish**, poultry, **eggs**, most dairy products, and most **grains** and pulses) produces acidic residues which need to be eliminated. Excess acidity in body tissues (acidosis) can result in metabolic and respiratory problems, and cause many diseases from arthritis to colds and infections. Severe acidosis can occur in diabetes and kidney disease. Excess alkalinity (alkalosis) is quite rare; it can result from taking too many antacid drugs or because of frequent vomiting.

Since alkalinity neutralizes acidity, in conditions of mild acidity, the balance can be restored by a diet containing plenty of alkaline foods. Most fruits and vegetables are alkalizing, as are **soybeans**, lima beans, millet and **buckwheat**. **Milk** is neutral. Among the most alkaline-forming foods are **figs**, **carrots**, **celery** and **pineapple**.

ACIDOPHILUS, LACTOBACILLUS

Intestinal bacteria (flora), which are the 'friendly' bacteria living in the gut, are vital for the proper absorption of nutrients; they also inhibit the growth of the candida albicans yeast (thrush). The *Lactobacillus acidophilus* bacteria are abundant in **yogurts** and serve to strengthen the intestinal flora. They can alleviate, and even prevent, a wide range of conditions, including intestinal putrefaction (food decaying in the intestines), vaginal yeast infections, constipation and flatulence. Their main antagonists are **antibiotics**, which kill all micro-organisms, whether 'friend' or 'foe'. Thus, when on antibiotics, it is very important to replenish the flora by eating plenty of yogurt and by supplementing with acidophilus capsules.

AGAR, AGAR-AGAR

A gelatinous substance produced from certain species of Japanese **seaweeds**, especially the *Gelidium* variety. Agar is unaffected by **enzymes** and, since seaweed is rich in **minerals** and **vitamins**, it provides an important source of nutrients. It is often used as a stabilizing agent (E406) in ice cream and other foods, and has traditionally been used by the Japanese as a form of gelatin. As such, agar is superior to the animal-derived gelatins in that it contains no **calories**, has a firmer texture and does not easily melt. It is available from health food shops as either flakes or bars, and dissolves readily in boiling water. It is easily digestible, making it particularly beneficial for sick people and children, and, due to its ability to absorb water and increase in bulk, it is also useful as a laxative. (See also CARRAGEENAN.)

AGRIMONY (*AGRIMONIA EUPATORIA*)

A perennial herb that grows wild in Northern Europe, it has astringent and anti-inflammatory properties and contains tannins which can tone the mucous membranes of the gut. Prepared as a herbal **tea** or infusion, it can have a very beneficial effect on the digestive organs – stomach, intestines, gallbladder and liver – and can also alleviate inflammation of the intestines caused by food irritants or infection (enteritis). As an infusion, it can be used as a gargle for treating mouth infections and is also helpful in the treatment of diarrhoea. Available from herbalists and health food stores.

ALCOHOL

Although the consumption of alcoholic beverages has been central to the social rituals of mankind throughout recorded history, nutritionally, alcohol has little to recommend it. As with **wine** and **beer**, if consumed in moderation, particularly in a social setting, it can add to the pleasure of the occasion and thereby reduce stress. However, it can become addictive and, consumed to excess, alcohol has extremely detrimental effects on the body's metabolism.

The alcohol in beverages is produced by the fermentation of fruit sugars and, when this is metabolized by the body, it produces a harmful chemical called acetaldehyde. It is this that causes the well-known after- effects, or 'hangovers', that so often afflict drinkers. As in the case of refined sugar, alcohol can deplete the body of essential **B vitamins, vitamin C, vitamin K, zinc, magnesium** and **potassium**. Even moderate consumption of 3 units was recently found to increase the risk of breast cancer, while higher consumption can result in liver and brain damage, ruptured blood vessels, agglutinated blood, varicose veins, haemorrhoids, thrombosis, damage to the prostate gland and sterility. In the final months of pregnancy, alcohol is suspected to increase the risk of premature birth. Alcohol can also increase the possibility of developing age-related conditions such as heart attacks, cataracts and skin wrinkles, and psychological disorders such as anxiety, depression, mental retardation and distorted emotions.

Vitamin B1, niacin, **vitamin C** and the **amino acid cysteine** can be helpful in protecting the body from some of the harmful effects of alcohol, and cravings can be alleviated by nutritional supplementation. The Chinese herb **kudzu** as well as the amino acid L-**glutamine** can be effective in this way and both are available in health food shops. Sometimes, the craving can be due to hypoglycaemia (low blood sugar). This can be verified by a Glucose Tolerance Test **(GTT),** and in this case a suitable diet prescribed by a nutritionist can help.

ALDER (*ALNUS GLUTINOSA*)

A small tree which is found wild throughout the British Isles and Europe. Traditionally, infusions of the shredded bark can relieve constipation and stimulate **bile** secretion, which is necessary for the process of digestion. Decoctions (boiled and simmered teas) can be used to make poultices to ease rheumatic joints, while infusions of the leaves can be used to treat inflammations. Available from larger health food stores or herbalists.

ALFALFA (*MEDICAGO SATIVA*)

A legume, it is a member of the pea family and is widely grown in Europe, North and South America, Asia and Australia. The seeds and sprouts of the plant are an excellent source of **beta carotene** and many key nutrients. They are especially rich in **minerals (potassium, iron, phosphorus, magnesium and calcium)** and **vitamins B1, B3, B12, D, C, E and K).** The sprouts are widely available in supermarkets and health food shops and are popularly eaten in salads; they can also be used to make alfalfa **tea.** Alfalfa acts as a tonic, stimulant, appetizer and diuretic, and can assist in the relief of urinary disorders and the alleviation of water retention (oedema).

ALLERGY, FOOD

A food allergy is an abnormal immune-system reaction to a substance in food. Normally, when hostile substances enter the blood, the immune system promptly reacts by producing antibodies to engulf and destroy them. In allergic conditions, however, the immune system reacts with the same hostility to certain 'innocent' substances, releasing histamine. This can cause a wide variety of distressing symptoms, from a simple rash to headaches and hypertension.

The causes of allergies are not fully understood by science, although it is known that the **protein** parts of foods and dust can trigger allergies. Two common causes of food allergies are low levels of stomach acid and a shortage of certain pancreatic digestive **enzymes**. The pancreas secretes enzymes which break down protein into its components, the **amino acids**. A shortage of these enzymes can result in partly digested protein, and it is these protein fragments that can induce food allergies in the intestines which produce not only physical, but also mental, symptoms.

Some common food additives, such as **benzoic acid** (E210) and tartrazine (E102) are known to cause allergic reactions in people with sensitivities, especially children.

The most common allergenic foods are cow's **milk, eggs, chocolate, oranges, wheat,** cheese, **tomatoes**, beef and maize, while among the least allergenic foods are **rice, peas** and **avocados**. A craving for a specific food can signal a food allergy, and the detection of these allergy-causing foods can be done by the 'pulse test' (see *Complete Nutrition*).

A number of nutrients can alleviate or cure these allergies, including **vitamin C** and **quercetin,** both potent antihistamines, **vitamin B6, zinc, vitamin E** and

calcium. In fact, some nutritionists believe that allergies may be caused by nutrient deficiencies.

ALMOND (*PRUNUS DULCIS*)

Used historically as food and medicine, almonds are a rich source of nutrients. They are 20 per cent protein and contain **vitamin E, calcium, magnesium, potassium, iron** and **zinc**. High in **fat** (up to 60 per cent), they are an excellent source of monounsaturated and polyunsaturated oils. Consequently, almonds have been shown to lower total **cholesterol** and to have an anti-cancer effect. Valued in traditional Indian medicine (**ayurveda**), almonds can help relieve phlegm, alleviate coughs and lubricate the intestines. Prepared as a drink (almond milk) by soaking them overnight in water, peeling off the brown skin and then blending the nuts with water in a blender, they make baby food. A few raw almonds can help alleviate heart burn. Almond oil is mainly used for cosmetic purposes.

ALOE VERA

A perennial plant indigenous to tropical areas of the Far East, southern Africa and the West Indies, it is now cultivated in some of the arid states of the USA, and is also grown in many places as a decorative plant. Nutritionally and medicinally, the plant is useful for the thick juice of its long leaves which has strong anti-fungal and anti-bacterial properties.

The aloe vera juice contains many important **vitamins** and **minerals**, as well as **beta carotene, enzymes, amino**

acids and the complex carbohydrate mucopolysaccharide. These are responsible for its many healing actions, which include the soothing of inflammations of the digestive tract and the relief of constipation, flatulence and the symptoms of irritable bowel syndrome (IBS). The gelatinous juice of the fresh leaves can also be used externally. It is reputed to heal wounds and can also be rubbed on the skin to alleviate sunburns, wrinkles, skin irritations and minor cuts. Infusions are good for bathing wounds and eyes. The juice has a somewhat repellent taste so, when taken orally, it is usually blended with fruit juice to make it more palatable. Pure American aloe vera juice is now readily available in most health foods shops.

ALUMINIUM

Everyday sources of this toxic element are processed cheeses, **baking soda**, antacid tablets, table **salt** and antiperspirants (E173). It can also be ingested through the use of aluminium cookware and utensils. Aluminium disturbs the calcium-phosphorus balance and causes the loss of **vitamin B1** and excesses of aluminium salts, which can accumulate in the brain and are implicated in memory loss, presenile dementia and Alzheimer's disease. **Vitamin C** is recommended to counteract the build up of these salts in the body, as is **garlic, seaweeds** and **wheat grass**.

AMARANTH (*AMARANTHUS HYPOCHONDRIACUSA*)

This grain is also known as Inca **wheat** and was the main staple of the Aztec diet due to its high **protein** content. It is now cultivated commercially in the American Midwest and is incorporated into some breakfast cereals. The crimson flowers have an astringent property and infusions of these can be effective in the treatment of diarrhoea and dysentery; they can also be used to reduce excessive menstrual bleeding. Amaranth is normally sold as a prepared cereal, but the flowers are also obtainable from some herbalists.

AMASAKE

A naturally processed sweetener of the macrobiotic range, which is becoming increasingly popular. Amasake is a fermented sweet **rice**, produced by cooking the whole rice grain in **water** with koji, a starter treated with a special yeast culture, *Aspergillus oryzae*, which converts the starch in the rice into simpler sugars. By the end of the fermentation stage, amasake resembles a thick rice pudding with a subtly balanced sweetness. Amasake is rich in maltose, but its sugars are not as refined or concentrated as **honey**.

Being derived from whole rice, amasake is also nourishing.

AMINO ACIDS

Amino acids are the building blocks of **proteins**. They are made up of a nitrogen-containing group, known as the amino group (NH2), and a carboxyl group containing carbon, oxygen and hydrogen (COOH). Specific amino acids may also contain **sulphur** and **iron** and, to create the many forms of protein in the body, the amino acids link together into the various chain structures (peptides) that give each kind of protein – whether in bone, hair, nails or blood – its specific characteristics. The formation of these proteins is governed by other proteins, the **nucleic acids** DNA and RNA, often described as the genetic blueprint of the body. DNA contains the master code and RNA conveys its instructions to cells where different kinds of proteins are formed. Protein synthesis is vitally important for sustaining life as cells are constantly being broken down and must be recreated.

Of the 24 known amino acids that make up the thousands of differing protein combinations, eight of these – **leucine, isoleucine, valine, methionine, threonine, lysine, phenylalanine** and **tryptophan** – are known as the 'essential amino acids' as all eight must be present simultaneously in the diet, and in the right proportions, in order to form what is termed 'complete protein'. None of these can be synthesized by the human body for itself and must be acquired from food. If even one is absent, or in a disproportionately low ratio to the others, then protein synthesis is halted or reduced. In this case, what is termed 'incomplete protein' results. This can happen in the diets of strict **vegetarians** or **vegans** subsisting on 'incomplete' vegetable protein, as it is the animal foods such as **meat, fish, eggs** and dairy produce that contain all the 'essentials' and form 'complete protein'. Individual free amino acids have been found to have specific beneficial effects, such as burning off fat, treating baldness, building muscle or relieving stress and, as such, they can be used as nutritional supplements. Some amino acids such as **arginine**, which are not adequately produced in many people, are considered 'semi-essential'.

ANGELICA (*ANGELICA ARCHANGELICA*)

Angelica is a large aromatic plant native to Northern Europe and Asia, which can be either biennial or perennial. It is found in damp places such as river banks and is also cultivated. For nutritional and medicinal purposes, the useful parts of the plant are its roots and seeds.

Angelica **tea**, produced from both the roots and the seeds, will aid digestion, relieve flatulence and stimulate **appetite**. It is useful for a number of digestive problems, including ulcers, vomiting and colic. Applied externally as a lotion, angelica can help relieve rheumatic pain and gout. A decoction of the root can be applied to the skin to treat scabies or itching.

An infusion can be made by adding half a cup of boiling water to one teaspoon of crushed seeds and steeping; a decoction can be made by boiling one teaspoon of crushed root in three-quarters of a cup of water, and then steeping for five minutes.

For convenience, angelica is sold as a liquid extract by some herbalists and the larger health food stores. This can be taken in a dosage of 10–30 drops in liquid, three times daily.

Caution: Angelica must not be taken by diabetics as it tends to elevate **blood sugar** levels.

ANISE, ANISEED (*PIMPINELLA ANISUM*)

Anise is an aromatic plant native to the Mediterranean regions, but is also cultivated. Its sweet seeds are used in Mediterranean cooking, mainly for flavouring.

As an infusion, anise helps digestion, relieves flatulence, improves **appetite** and alleviates cramps, nausea and colic in children. As a tisane, anise can be used to stimulate milk production in nursing mothers and an infusion of the seeds is reputed to bring on delayed menstruation.

A tisane is made by boiling half a teaspoon of crushed seed in half a pint of **water** and straining it. An infusion is made with one teaspoon of crushed seed boiled with a cup of **water** and allowed to steep for 10 minutes.

Anise is also known to promote energy circulation and increase the metabolic rate, which is valuable in any weight-loss programme. Available from larger health food stores and herbalists.

ANTACIDS

Antacid drugs bring only temporary relief, not a permanent cure, and, unless prescribed, anyone using antacids should realize that the symptoms of too much acid in the stomach are similar to those of having too little. In the latter case, therefore, taking antacids will only serve to exacerbate the problem. In addition, some antacids contain **aluminium**, a toxic element which can build up in the body and give rise to an array of disorders.

Heartburn resulting from low acidity in the stomach can be relieved with **betaine HCl** tablets. In fact, since stomach secretions are known to diminish with age, some authorities recommend that anyone over 40 should use a HCl supplement with each main meal.

In some cases, digestive **enzymes** such as **pancreatin tablets** can help, but correct **food combinations** are considered to be the simplest and most effective way of preventing stomach over-acidity, heartburn and dyspepsia.

For quick relief, taking 2–3 **dolomite** tablets with each meal is best. In the author's experience, a glass of cold **milk** or a few raw **almonds** can be very effective in cases of heartburn. Another simple way to avoid heartburn is to drink fluids before meals, rather than after, as this dilutes gastric juices.

ANTIBIOTICS

Once thought to eradicate all infectious diseases, the use of antibiotics is beginning to decline. While sensitivities to the drugs are on the increase, their actual effectiveness in treatments has decreased. Several strains of bacteria have developed immunity and resist antibiotic treatments. It is now estimated that 20 per cent of infections contracted in hospitals fail to respond to antibiotic treatment, and in the USA alone more than 100,000 people die each year from such infections.

Originally, antibiotics were very powerful and their use in emergencies saved many lives. Unfortunately, doctors developed a tendency to prescribe antibiotics indiscriminately and eventually, as a result of overuse, many bacteria developed resistance to the drugs and it became necessary to prescribe higher and higher doses. In time, a vicious circle was formed as the higher doses created stronger side-effects.

Since antibiotics are unable to distinguish between micro-organisms, they kill the 'friendly' intestinal bacteria (flora) needed for food absorption along with the pathogenic bacteria. One of the results of this has been a proliferation of vaginal yeast infections in women who have been prescribed tetracyclines. Antibiotics can also neutralize the effects of the contraceptive pill. As a result, doctors are now reserving the use of antibiotics as a last resort, and there is a growing tendency to prepare patients for surgery by fortifying their immune system over a period of time with balanced, well-supplemented diets.

ANTIDEPRESSANTS, NUTRITIONAL

Nutritional treatment of depression, stress and anxiety can include two of the **amino acids**: DLPA (DL-phenylalanine), which increases levels of noradrenaline and **dopamine** in the brain, and **GABA** (gamma-aminobutyric acid), which is gaining popularity for its anti-anxiety effects. The latter is derived in the body from **glutamic acid** and acts as an inhibitory neurotransmitter. That is, it slows down the frantic activity of the nerve cells in the brain's lymbic system, which is the body's emotional alarm bell.

Calcium is a well-known calming mineral which can even alleviate insomnia if taken at bedtime at doses of 500 mg. Helpful **vitamins** for treating stress and depression are **vitamin C** and the **B vitamins**, expecially **B1**, niacin and **pantothenic acid**, while beneficial herbs include **hawthorn, kava kava, linden, St John's wort** and **valerian.**

Among the foods that can acerbate depression and anxiety and should be avoided are white sugar, white flour, **caffeine** and a high-fat diet. Similarly, **alcohol** consumption and smoking should be reduced or cut out completely.

ANTIOXIDANTS

Antioxidants are substances that neutralize free radicals. These are atoms or molecules that are formed during food metabolism, or by pollutants, smoking and radiation, and are electronically unbalanced. In stable molecules, electrons come in pairs, but free radicals have unpaired electrons – either one is missing or there is an extra one – and to restabilize themselves they grab an electron from another molecule. In this way, another free radical is created and a destructive chain reaction is begun or continued.

Free radicals, unless or until they are neutralized, damage various body cells. For instance, they can distort the **DNA** genetic blueprint, thus causing many of the degenerative diseases of ageing, such as heart disease, cancer and strokes; they also attack blood vessels, producing blood clots and atherosclerosis, and they can damage brain cells, creating memory loss and senility.

The antioxidants serve as free radical scavengers, neutralizing and defending the body from their oxidative damage. The body protects itself with various antioxidant **enzymes,** such as superoxide dismutase **(SOD)** and catalase or **glutathione** peroxide. Free radicals are also neutralized by antioxidant nutrients such as the **vitamins A, C, E, B1, B5, B6**, niacin and **PABA**, the **amino acid cysteine** (found in **eggs**), **minerals zinc** and **selenium,** catechols (found in bananas and **potatoes**), phenolics (found in **grapes** and other fruits), **quercetin** (found in **onion** and **garlic**), **rutin** (found in **buckwheat**) and hesperidin (found in citrus rind). Other foods high in natural antioxidants include **wheat grass**, berries and dark green vegetables. (See also BIOFLAVONOIDS.)

Polyphenols are a large class of powerful antioxidant micronutrients, which are present in most plants, spices, herbs, seeds, dark berries, fruits and vegetables. Typical examples are resveratrol in red grapes or capsaicin in chilli and paprika. Their molecules consist of multiple phenols (C6 H5 OH), mostly made up of 6–Ring tannins (like the ones used in leather tanning). Due to their strong antioxidant effect, polyphenols protect from UV light and help prevent degenerative diseases such as cancer and cardiovascular disease.

Commercially, chemical antioxidants such as BHA (E320) and BHT (E321) are used as preservatives in processed foods, to prevent spoilage and colour change. Prolonged consumption of BHA and BHT can be harmful to the kidneys.

APPETITE

For anyone wishing to reduce weight, or needing to curb their appetite for other reasons, the following nutrients can be helpful if included in the diet: **avocados, bran** and fibrous foods, **celery** stalks, **guar gum**, hydroxycitric acid (HCA) as in Citrimax tablets, together with the amino acid L-**phenylalanine**, and also freshly squeezed **lemon** juice.

For those needing to stimulate their appetite, the following foods are recommended: **alfalfa sprouts, apples, carrot** juice, **cayenne pepper, celery** leaves, chicken, **cider vinegar, corn, grapefruit**, liver, **mushrooms, oranges, strawberries** and **tomatoes**. In addition, herbs such as **agrimony, anise** and **camomile**, together with the **vitamin B complex, zinc** and **brewer's yeast** are also useful.

APPLES (*MALUS*)

Apples are a highly nutritious and cleansing fruit, as well as a good source of **vitamins A** and **B1**; they are also rich in a number of minerals including **potassium, calcium, phosphorus** and **sodium**, and the bioflavonoid **quercetin**.

In addition, they contain malic and tartaric acids, which inhibit gastric fermentation and bacteria proliferation in the digestive tract. In fact, a Cornell University study showed that apple extracts can significantly reduce the risk of colon cancer. An average apple weighs 140 g and contains about 80 calories and 5 g of dietary fibre.

The fruit are rich in **pectin**, which has numerous uses: it can help reduce high **cholesterol** levels and remove toxic metals such as **lead** and **mercury** from the body; it is very beneficial for intestinal problems and it binds radioactive residues and excretes them from the body It is also used as a stabilizer (E440b) in the commercial production of foods such as jams and preserves.

Apples can help cleanse the lungs of phlegm and protect them from smoking; they also boost immunity and stimulate the **appetite**. In addition, apple juice is very cleansing for the liver and gall bladder.

APRICOTS (*PRUNUS ARMENIACA*)

Originating from China, apricots are a popular seasonal fruit which ripen in June and July. Ripe apricots are an excellent source of **vitamins A** and **potassium**. A serving of 100 g contains over 80 g of vitamin A. Apricots are recommended eating in cases of lung conditions. They are also high in **copper** and **cobalt** and can therefore be beneficial in the treatment of anaemia. In addition, they contain substantial amounts of **calcium**, **silicon**, **phosphorus** and **vitamin C**.

Caution: Apricots should be used cautiously during pregnancy and avoided in cases of diarrhoea.

ARACHIDONIC ACID (*AA*)

It is one of the essential fatty acids, which have numerous duties, and cause the production of prostaglandins (PG) of the type PGE2. These are hormone-like compounds which stimulate and control many bodily functions. PGE2 accelerates **blood clotting** and increases water retention, but excesses of it, which arise primarily from consumption of animal products, can cause pain and inflammation. AA also releases leukotrienes; these are substances which can help to heal wounds and injuries but, in excess, will stimulate such conditions as breast lumps and arthritis, especially rheumatoid arthritis, asthma, psoriasis and lupus erythematosus. **Aspirin** and steroid drugs inhibit the synthesis of PGE2 and can therefore reduce blood clotting, pain and fever. Indeed, aspirin is now widely used to protect vulnerable people from heart attacks. However, as it also inhibits PGE1, which counteracts the action of PGE2, a better choice is to increase the level of PGE1, which has a natural anti–inflammatory action. This can be done by taking **evening primrose oil** and excluding animal foods (except for some **fish**).

ARGININE (*L-ARGININE*)

Arginine is a semi–essential **amino acid** which, with its derivative **ornithine**, stimulates the secretion by the pituitary gland of **growth hormone** in the brain. This is essential not only for children's growth, but also for adults, since it promotes repair of worn tissues and helps to heal wounds. In addition, it stimulates the growth of T-lymphocytes – immune cells that identify, engulf and destroy invading bacteria and carcinogenic chemicals. In this respect, arginine can be extremely useful in the treatment of autoimmune diseases such as arthritis and multiple sclerosis. Arginine and **ornithine** have also been reported to stimulate weight loss and increase sperm count and motility. Supplemental arginine can raise nitric oxide levels, a compound that increases blood flow and facilitates penile erection.

Arginine is usually taken in doses of 2–4 g on an empty stomach, preferably at bed time, as peak secretion of growth hormones are released after falling asleep, or one hour before strenuous exercise.

Caution: Arginine and ornithine should not be used by children or pregnant and lactating women. Arginine is contra-indicated in herpes.

ARNICA (*ARNICA MONTANA*)

A perennial plant, also known as mountain tobacco, it grows in the mountainous regions of Europe, Siberia, northern Asia and the western United States and Canada. It has been widely used for centuries as a healing herb, especially for bruising and trauma in cases of accident or injury. However, it should never be used on broken skin or open wounds.

An infusion prepared from the root will stimulate perspiration and help to reduce temperature in a feverish cold; it can also be used to soothe inflamed mucous membranes and nasal passages, and act as a diuretic and general stimulant. Infusions can also be applied externally as a hair tonic. Available from larger health food stores and herbalists.

AROMATHERAPY

This is an ancient art which uses aromatic plant essences which, although not oily in texture, are known as essential oils. These can be extracted from the flowers, leaves, stems, fruits, seeds and/or roots of the plants, and their effects are many and varied. As inhalations or applied to the skin, these essential oils can be used to relieve physical conditions, restore mental and physical balance, and create a feeling of well-being.

Aromatic herbs have been used for thousands of years for both healing and cosmetic purposes. For instance, ancient **Ayurvedic** texts include aromatic essences in many of their treatments, but modern aromatherapy was rediscovered in the 1920s by René-Maurice Gattefossé, a French chemist, who studied the therapeutic effects of essential oils after accidentally discovering the beneficial effects of **lavender** oil in the treatment of burns.

More recently, with the resurgence of interest in natural living and complementary medicines, aromatherapy has become increasingly popular. Around three thousand essential oils are used by trained aromatherapists, most of whom use a holistic approach, i.e. they do not treat merely the symptom, but consider the complete physical and emotional state as an entity. An essential oil may contain many different compounds, all working together to provide benefit. Many aromatherapy blends are available which are carefully balanced to produce specific effects such as relaxation, sensuality, clarity and inspiration. For example, a sensual blend can be made from ylang ylang, lavender and sandalwood, while premenstrual tension can be eased with a blend of clary, **sage** and geranium. Essential oils are quickly absorbed, and inhalation is very effective for delivering the active ingredients to the bloodstream. Many essential oils are also very effective as antimicrobial and antifungal agents.

ARTICHOKE (*CYNARA SCOLYMUS*)

A large, thistle-like perennial plant which originated in the Mediterranean region and was traditionally used by ancient Greeks and Romans as a remedy for digestive disorders, the globe artichoke is now widely cultivated in temperate climates. The flower heads are commonly eaten as vegetables but extracts of leaves and roots were once used to treat liver disorders, jaundice and atherosclerosis. Artichokes provide a number of **vitamins** and **minerals**, and one of their key active ingredients, cynarin, was shown by clinical studies to stimulate **bile** flow from the gall bladder, thus mobilising fatty stores and reducing **cholesterol**. Other studies found that artichoke extracts can help digestive complaints such as poor appetite, nausea and abdominal discomfort.

ASCORBIC ACID SEE VITAMIN C

ASPARAGINE

This is a non-essential **amino acid** which, with **glutamic acid**, is most commonly found in the brain. It is thought to regulate brain and nerve metabolism, and is used in the treatment of mental and emotional disorders. Available from health food stores.

ASPARAGUS (*ASPARAGUS OFFICINALIS*)

A nutritious green vegetable, it is a perennial that originated in the Mediterranean region and in Africa. It grows best in moderate climates and the young shoots, which are mainly used in cooking, are a rich source of **vitamins** and **minerals**. It is especially rich in **vitamin E** and 2 oz can provide a good daily dose. Asparagus contains **asparagine**, an **amino acid**, which has calming properties. The plant is also a diuretic and can aid the elimination of water through urination, a special boon in cases of water retention (oedema). Asparagus can be used to treat many kidney conditions, but it should not be used in cases of inflammations. It is also helpful in cleansing **cholesterol** from arteries and hence is useful in treating vascular problems such as hypertension and arteriosclerosis.

Caution: In excessive amounts, asparagus can irritate the kidneys.

ASPARTAME

This is a popular artificial sweetener used widely in diet products, from soft drinks to cereals, but also sold as a tabletop sweetener for **tea** and coffee under such brand names as Nutrasweet or Equal. Made up of aspartic acid, **phenylalanine** and methanol, aspartame is 180 times sweeter than sugar and lacks the bitter aftertaste of saccharin. It is unsuitable for use in cooking because its flavour is changed when heated.

Phenylalanine, an **amino acid** component of aspartame, poses a problem for people with phenylketonuria (PKU), a congenital hereditary condition caused by the body's inability to oxidise phenylalanine to **tyrosine** due to a defective enzyme. Such people risk brain damage if they use aspartame and that is why Nutrasweet diet products carry the warning 'contains phenylalanine.' Although no serious adverse effects were documented, a small segment of the population is known to be sensitive to aspartame. High intake of aspartame through excessive use of diet sodas is claimed to cause complaints such as headaches, nausea, dizziness or irritabilty, probably by overconsumption of phenylalanine and methanol.

ASPARTIC ACID

A non–essential **amino acid**, it has chelating effects – that is, it can bind toxic elements such as **lead** and **mercury**, and assist in their excretion from the body. Aspartic acid, with **phenylalanine**, produces the popular artificial sweetener

aspartame, which is 180 times sweeter than sugar and is used mainly in diet soft drinks and sweetening tablets.

ASPIRIN

Aspirin is an anti-inflammatory drug originally isolated from willow bark which is readily obtainable over-the-counter and has become widely used as an inexpensive painkiller. It is commonly used to treat the aches and pains of conditions such as migraine and arthritis. However, aspirin is not a cure; it can only mitigate or alleviate pain and, in spite of its popularity and being freely available, it is not totally harmless. Not only does it deplete the body's supply of **vitamin C**, large or frequent dosing with aspirin can irritate the stomach and cause stomach haemorrhages and ulcers.

In recent years, aspirin has been widely prescribed in the treatment of arthritis and to protect from heart disease, as it is known to block the production of PGE2, a prostaglandin. This is a hormone-like compound and excesses of it can increase **bloodclotting** and contribute to heart attack. However, aspirin also inhibits PGE1 and PGE3, which are beneficial prostaglandins that counteract the effects of PGE2. A preferable choice of treatment, therefore, is to increase the body's levels of PGE1 by using supplements such as **evening primrose oil** while, at the same time, reducing the intake of animal foods.

ASTRAGALUS (ASTRAGALUS MAMBRANACEUS)

A traditional Chinese herb, its root was found to increase resistance to disease by fortifying the immune system. For example, it increases the body's secretion of interferon, which fights viruses. According to Chinese studies, astragalus reduces susceptibility to colds and their duration. Astragalus is indicated, together with **echinacea** and **ginseng**, for use in the degenerative conditions of ageing such as heart disease, cancer and arthritis. Since it is a diuretic, astragalus can be useful to reduce water retention (oedema). During the past decade, astragalus has been 'discovered' by Western science, and is increasingly being incorporated into nutritional formulas sold in health food shops.

AUBERGINE (*SOLANUM MELONGENA*)

Originating in China and brought over to Europe in the Middle Ages, aubergine, also known as eggplant, is a non-starchy fruit which combines well with other foods as a versatile ingredient in casseroles, dips and salads. It is high in dietary **fibre**, low in fat and contains an array of nutrients such as **vitamins A, B1, B3, B6, folic acid**, and the minerals **iron, calcium, magnesium, copper, manganese, phosphorus** and especially **potassium**. It is also rich in anthocyanin flavonoids, particularly one called nasunin, a potent antioxidant and free-radical scavenger known to protect the cell membranes, whose integrity is crucial for proper metabolic activity and general health. In addition, the mucilaginous fibre of aubergine can help to lower **cholesterol** levels, while its potassium content is useful in the prevention of water retention.

Aubergine is reputed to reduce bleeding and has traditionally been used for the treatment of haemorrhoids and bleeding in general. It is an astringent food and is useful in the treatment of diarrhoea. It is also very suitable for inclusion in weight loss programmes as one cup of cooked cubes contains only 27

calories, 3 mg of **sodium** and a trace of fat, but, due to its high fibre content, it provides a feeling of fullness. It is best bought fresh when it is firm, weighty, and free of scars and cuts.

AVOCADO (*PERSEA AMERICANA*)

Native to Mexico, Guatemala and other Central and South American countries, avocados are now grown in many tropical and subtropical regions, particularly in Florida and California.

Containing an abundance of **vitamins** and **minerals**, avocados are particularly rich in **vitamins E, A and B** and **potassium**. One avocado has the potassium content of two **bananas**. Avocados are an excellent source of monounsaturated fatty acids, second only to olives. They contain about 20 per cent **fat**, and their oils include oleic and linoleic acid, which can help lower **cholesterol** levels. Avocados provide an excellent source of nutritious **protein** and are often recommended for nursing mothers. As an oily fruit, avocado is a good internal lubricator, and can be used to soothe stomach and duodenal ulcers. It is also known to beautify the skin.

Avocado is rich in **lecithin**, a fat emulsifier which promotes brain function, and most of its calorific value (80 per cent) comes from easily digested fat. It is very beneficial for hypoglycaemics (people with low **blood sugar** levels) as it contains mannoheptulose, a special type of sugar which depresses the secretion of insulin; thus, in contrast to white sugar, it helps stabilize proper blood sugar levels. For this reason, avocados can be a valuable contribution to weight loss programmes since they help to satisfy hunger for longer periods of time. Avocados are also a useful ingredient for correct **food-combining** diets, as

they combine well with both proteins and starches. Just one
100 g serving (about half an avocado) provides 160 calories,
2 g protein, 8.5 g carbohydrates, 6.7 g fibre and 14.7 g fat. Of
this, 9.8 g is monounsaturated fat, 2.8 g polyunsaturated fat
and only 2.1 g is saturated fat.

AYURVEDA

A traditional Indian approach to healthy living and
longevity, ayurveda means 'Science of Life.' With more and
more ayurvedic formulas sold in health food stores,
ayurveda is increasingly becoming a Western alternative
medicine modality. First mentioned in ancient Sanscrit
texts, it is a complete natural health care system, treating
both body and mind, using various healing therapies to
ensure and maintain health and well-being and, ultimately,
to reach a state of bliss. Ayurveda is thus the first holistic
system of diagnosis and treatment, integrating nutrition,
herbalism, meditation and awareness.

Ayurvedic medicine uses complex herbal and mineral
formulations to restore the balance of every bodily
function, preferably before minor imbalances become diseases.
Sometimes, this preventive approach is reinforced to cure
a fully developed disease. But even then, ayurveda aims at
restoring the power of the body to heal itself, thus ensuring
that the treatment is effective and permanent. In
doing so, ayurveda treats first the patient, not just the
symptoms. Ayurvedic medicines include formulations
consisting of plants and **minerals** in fixed, precise proportions
according to a vast pharmacopoea.

B

BABIES, FOOD

It is most important to breast feed for the baby's first six months at least, if at all possible. The mother's milk (colostrum) in the first few days after delivery is rich in antibodies and lymphocytes, which boost the immunity of the child to diseases. Once established, breast feeding largely determines the baby's health, not only in the first few months but for many years to come, and saves needless miseries such as ear infections, colic and allergies. Research has shown that the substitution of cow's **milk** in the early months can be correlated with later obesity and heart disease. It would seem that the high **cholesterol** level in a mother's milk – as opposed to low cholesterol in cow's milk – serves in fact to establish lower cholesterol levels in later years. Recent studies have also indicated that when cow's milk is introduced before four months of age, this may trigger the autoimmune process and increase the risk of diabetes developing in later years (see *Complete Nutrition*)

From the age of six months, mashed vegetables and other foods should be introduced gradually, while at the same time decreasing the consumption of milk. Then, when the first molar appears – usually at about 18 months – this is a sign that the pancreatic **enzymes** in the intestines are ready to synthesize more solid foods. Of course, this is only a general timetable and every baby is different: some can be weaned at a very early age while others will refuse weaning even after the first birthday. When mother's milk is not available it is advisable to use either the milk from another mother (a wet nurse) or goat's milk, or a combination of both. Babies born to **vegan** mothers are known to thrive on **almond** milk or soya milk.

BACTERIA, INTESTINAL SEE PROBIOTICS

BAKING SODA

Baking soda (sodium bicarbonate) is an alkaline leavening agent. When kneaded into the acidic bread dough before baking, it creates a reaction which releases bubbles of carbon dioxide causing the dough to "rise." Its big advantage over slow-acting yeast is that baking soda works instantly. Soda bread is now becoming increasingly popular as more people with a variety of symptoms ranging from indigestion to headaches, find out that they are allergic to baker's yeast. Baking soda, however, depletes two B vitamins, **thiamine (B1)** and **folic acid** – and neutralizes **vitamin C**. Some brands of baking soda include **aluminium salts** such as sodium–aluminate–sulphate (E-521), which can accumulate in the brain, causing memory loss and dementia. Sourdough bread is a better alternative. It is leavened with a fermented "starter", a culture of naturally occurring airborne yeast and lactobacilli, which ferments the dough and leavens it. Sourdough bread is now available in more grocery stores, but can also be baked at home with a home-made starter, prepared by mixing a bit of wheat flour with water, keeping it wet and allowing it to ferment for 2–3 days. Baking soda is also a useful dentifrice which can help whiten teeth and neutralize acidic plaque. Half a teaspoon of baking soda dissolved in a glass of water can help relieve heartburn.

Caution: Baking soda should not be used as an antacid by people on low-**sodium** diets.

BALM, LEMON BALM (*MELISSA OFFICINALIS*)

A perennial plant, originally native to the eastern
Mediterranean, it can now be found growing wild
throughout most of Europe, and is cultivated mainly as a
culinary herb for its lemon-scented leaves. An infusion of
the leaves can be used to dull pain, ease toothache, and
relieve flatulence, cramps, indigestion and colic. Since it
increases perspiration, it is useful in treating colds by
reducing feverishness. Traditionally, it has been used to treat
nervousness, depression and insomnia, and it is also claimed
to stimulate the onset of menstruation and relieve period
pains. The leaves can be used to prepare a pleasant, aromatic
tea with soothing and relaxing properties. Available from
larger health food stores and herbalists.

BANANA (*MUSA*)

An aromatic fruit, which originated in Asia, it is now grown
in the hot, damp climates of tropical and sub-tropical countries.
Bananas are rich in **potassium** and low in **sodium**:
an average-size banana contains a whopping 440 mg potassium
and only 1 mg sodium. As such, bananas are used to treat
hypertension and detoxify the body. Their principal aroma is
amyl acetate and they contain large amounts of **tryptophan**,
an amino acid that is converted to **serotonin**, an inhibiting
brain neurotransmitter which makes bananas a calming food,
especially when taken with **milk** before bedtime.

Bananas serve as a good internal lubricator for the
intestines as they moisten dryness and, although they are
commonly given to children, they are suitable for everyone,
especially for people who tend to suffer from hypertension,

weak digestion and general weakness. Bananas are astringent before fully ripened, which makes them useful in the treatment of diarrhoea and haemorrhoids. When fully ripe, bananas can be beneficial in the treatment of constipation and ulcers.

Traditionally, the African Zulus used to rub banana peels on their skins as a tribal medicine for any skin condition. Modern resarch has found that banana peel rubbed on the red, scaly patches of psoriasis can provide relief without the side-effects of conventional treatments. The active ingredients in banana peels, the esterified fatty acids, have been isolated and incorporated in to a patented lotion, Exorex Lotion, which is now being marketed.

BARBERRY (*BERBERIS VULGARIS*)

The common barberry is a deciduous shrub that grows wild throughout Europe and the eastern United States. Both its roots and berries can be used in infusions. An infusion of the root promotes the secretion of bile and is therefore beneficial in liver disorders. The bark of the root has a laxative effect. Decoctions of either the root or berries make a good mouthwash or gargle for mouth and throat irritations. Available from herbalists.

Caution: Neither high nor low blood pressure should be treated with barberry.

BARLEY (*HORDEUM*)

Probably one of the first cultivated cereals, barley is grown in almost all the temperate regions of Europe and North America. It is a nutritious and easily digested cereal, providing a good source of **fibre, iron, calcium** and **protein**. It is known to strengthen the stomach and intestines and to soothe inflamed membranes, and is believed to help reduce tumours and oedema. It can be used in the alleviation of painful urination and as a mild laxative. Sprouted barley is even more nutritious and can help indigestion and abdominal bloating. It is also a strong blood purifier.

Barley grass, which can be grown at home, is richer in chlorophyll, **vitamin A** and **enzymes**, making it easier to digest. It also contains the antioxidant enzyme **SOD** and mucopolysaccharides which give it anti-inflammatory properties. Barley grass has a high protein content of 20 per cent, about the same as that of **meat**.

Barley malt is a sweetener prepared from sprouted barley. During sprouting, starch is converted to maltose, which does not harm teeth as sugar does and is therefore a much safer and more nutritious sweetener. Ground roasted barley is frequently used as an ingredient in several brands of coffee substitute and is recommended as a relief for fatigue. Available in health food shops.

BASIL (*OCIMUM BASILICUM*)

An annual with a pungent aroma, the plant is native to India but has been grown throughout the Mediterranean regions for thousands of years. It is now cultivated throughout southern and western Europe as an aromatic culinary herb. The leaves have **appetite**-stimulating properties and are generally used as a culinary flavouring. Infusions of the leaves can be used to relieve flatulence, fermentation, stomach cramps and constipation, and the plant is also said to relieve nausea. Available from supermarkets.

BAY LEAVES SEE LAUREL

BEANS SEE LEGUMES

BEARBERRY (*ARCTOSTAPHYLOS UVA-URSI*)

Bearberry, also called uva ursi, is an evergreen shrub of the *Ericaceae* family. It has small, bitter leaves and produces juicy but insipid berries. The leaves contain tannins, which are astringent, and glycosides, which are excellent antiseptics and anti-bacterial. Until the advent of **antibiotics**, bearberry was used as a urinary tract antiseptic. The astringent properties of the leaves can also be utilized in an infusion to help alleviate diarrhoea and bleeding. Bearberry also has diuretic properties and can be used to reduce uric acid levels, for the relief of pain caused by kidney stones and gravel, and for the alleviation of the symptoms of chronic cystitis. Available from larger health food stores and herbalists.

Caution: Excessive use of bearberry can cause stomach pain.

BEE POLLEN

Pollen is the yellowish dust produced by the anthers of male flowers. It is transferred by bees to the ovaries of the female flowers resulting in their fertilization and the development of fruit or seeds. Specific types of pollen are also collected by bees for storage in their hives as food for the young bees.

The composition of bee pollen varies according to the type of flower it has come from but, whatever its source, it is one the most nourishing foods available to mankind. On average, it contains 30 per cent **amino acids (protein)**, 50 per cent **carbohydrates**, 14 per cent polyunsaturated fatty acids, a large concentration of **minerals** and trace elements, many of the **A, C, D, E** and **B-complex vitamins** and **bioflavonoids**. The protein is complete and rates higher than meat in essential amino acids.

Nutritionally, it is so perfectly balanced that, in itself, it represents a complete survival food.

Bee pollen has been extensively studied for its beneficial effects. It has been given to athletes as it has been found to improve energy and endurance; in the Republic of Georgia, the consumption of bee pollen has been correlated with longevity. Bee pollen has also been found to prevent colds and flu, help the immune system to fight virus infections, relieve fatigue, improve **appetite**, increase sexual potency and fertility, alleviate painful menstruation, reduce the hot flushes of menopause for women and alleviate enlarged prostate in men.

Bee pollen is considerably less allergenic than wind-borne pollens. It should be taken regularly for at least one month: up to 20 g a day provides a normal supplement, while 40 g constitutes a therapeutic dosage. Available from larger health food stores.

BEER

Considered a low-alcohol recreational drink, beer is drunk socially in large quantities, more like a soda than an alcoholic drink.

Made from malted **barley**, flavoured with **hops** and brewed by slow fermentation, beer can contain anything from four to eight per cent alcohol. Therefore, large consumption of beer can easily become an alcohol abuse. Beer can also contain additional flavourings and additives, particularly caramel (E150), which gives many beers their colour.

Beers flavoured with hops contain small amounts of xanthohumol, a powerful antioxidant compound in hops that protects against heart disease and cancer. The amounts however, are too small to be preventative.

Perceptions of the safety of beer are conflicting and are expressed by both enthusiastic proponents and opponents. Sensible consumption seems to raise the level of the 'good' **HDL cholesterol** and helps prevent blockages in the heart arteries of healthy people. But do not rush to use beer to lower your high cholesterol: a famous German study revealed that the alcohol did not benefit people with existing high cholesterol. Several studies suggested that light beer drinkers have less heart disease than heavy drinkers. And **cobalt** added to beer to preserve its foam was shown to contribute to heart disease in heavy beer drinkers.

Heavy beer drinkers should remember that beer is also high in purines, digestive by-products that convert to uric acid, the build-up of which can bring on or worsen gout. Heavy beer drinking was found to increase the risk of rectal and lung cancer in men, and breast cancer in women. Higher alcohol consumption may also lead to cirrhosis of the liver, high blood pressure, varicose veins and haemorrhoids, heart irregularities, coronary thrombosis and foetal defects.

A study done in Finland in 1997 confirmed the danger of beer binges. Drinking six cans of beer a day increased fourfold the risk of cardiovascular disease compared to those who drank only one or two cans. In addition, a high rate of behavioural problems, such as aggressiveness and violence, were observed in beer bingers. No wonder that more brands

of non- or low-alcohol beer are now available. Practising
moderation in beer drinking seems to be good advice.

BEETROOT (*BETA VULGARIS*)

A vegetable originating from the Mediterranean region which
has long been used for its health benefits, beetroot is rich in
iron and also contains **vitamins B1, B2,** and **C** plus minerals
potassium, manganese, phosphorus and **silicone**. Its leaves
are rich in **beta carotene**. Traditionally, beetroot has been used
to detoxify the liver, purify the blood and improve circulation,
lowering the risk of heart attacks. Drinking one cup of beetroot
juice a day, was shown by one study to lower blood pressure
by about 7 per cent. Recent studies have revealed the reason
for these benefits. Beetroot is rich in dietary nitrates, which the
body converts to nitric oxide (NO), a gas that provides oxygen
to every cell of the body for optimal function. Nitric oxide is
a vasodilator – that is, it relaxes arteries, improves blood flow
and lowers blood pressure. This explains the potential ability
of beetroot to help prevent heart attacks, strokes, damage to
kidneys and poor circulation in legs. Physical fitness studies
found that beetroot juice increased energy and improved
athletic performance. Whole beets and juice are available from
supermarkets and grocers.

BELLADONA (*ATROPA BELLADONA*)

Commonly known as deadly nightshade, this poisonous
plant grows wild throughout Europe and many Asian
countries. It contains several alkaloids, including atropine,
which relieves asthma, hyoscyiamine, which induces sleep
and can cause paralysis, belladonine, which is a narcotic
and painkiller, and scopolamine, another painkiller which

reduces high blood pressure and produces twilight sleep.

Caution: The narcotic action of belladona affects the central nervous system and can cause paralysis. It is available on prescription in tinctures and extracts, and it should only be used under medical supervision.

BENZOIC ACID

A commonly used preservative (E210) in many processed foods, it is known to cause allergies in sensitive people. Children are especially vulnerable and allergic reactions can include hyperactivity, abdominal pains, diarrhoea, asthma and rashes. Saccharin is a derivative of benzoic acid.

BETA CAROTENE

Beta carotene is a **vitamin A** precursor (also called provitamin A) and one of the many plant pigments known collectively as **carotenoids**. It is the most prevalent cartenoid in plants. These plant pigments are potent **antioxidants**, protecting the plants from destruction by the free radicals generated by dangerous sun rays, and without these protective carotenoids the plants would quickly shrivel. People can acquire the same protection from antioxidants by eating foods high in beta carotene, such as **carrots**, sweet **potato**, cantaloupe, **pumpkin** and leafy green vegetables. The microalgae **spirulina** and dunaliella are among the highest sources of beta carotene.

Although beta carotene is converted to vitamin A in the body, it has additional biological properties of its own. It is a stronger antioxidant than vitamin A and studies have shown that it protects the body from several types of cancer, especially lung cancer. Beta carotene also acts as a filter, protecting the eye lens from cataract. In addition, it boosts the immune system and stimulates the T-cells, providing a strong protection to the thymus gland.

BETAINE HCL

This is a stomach acid supplement available in health food shops for people with low gastric secretion. A betaine HCl tablet taken after a meal can improve food tolerance and digestion, and its use can also help conditions resulting from low stomach acid, such as heartburn. Since low stomach acid is known to cause allergies, betaine HCl can also help reduce various allergy symptoms. Gastric secretions are known to be reduced with age and Dr Alan Nittler, author of *A New Breed of Doctor*, recommends that everyone over the age of 40 should take betaine HCl tablets as a matter of course.

BILBERRY (*VACCINIUM MYRTILLUS*)

Also known as whortleberry, this small perennial plant grows wild in the poor soil of sandy areas and moors and both its berries, which are black, and its leaves can be used for medicinal purposes. Bilberry is rich in flavonoids, particularly proanthocyanidins and anthocyanidins, both of which are powerful **antioxidants** and have an anti-inflammatory effect, strengthening capillaries and collagen. Bilberry extracts, which are rich in anthocyanidin compounds, are now increasingly used to treat eye conditions such as near-sightedness, and to improve night vision and reverse diabetic retinopathy. An infusion of the leaves is antiseptic and can be used to treat diarrhoea and dysentery; it can also act as a diuretic. Capsules and formulas for improving eyesight are available from larger health food stores.

BILE

A thick fluid secreted by the liver, bile is produced from **cholesterol** through the action of an enzyme and with the help of **vitamin C**. It is used by the duodenum to emulsify **fats** and assist with the absorption of fatty acids. Excess bile is stored in the gall bladder, where it is discharged into the duodenum as it is needed.

A high level of vitamin C in the diet helps to promote bile production, which, in turn, assists in the reduction of cholesterol levels. At the same time, dietary improvement can help to increase the production of bile since, when a diet is low in **protein** or high in sugar, little bile is produced. As a result of this, fats are poorly dissolved in the digestive tract and parts of the undissolved fats will then combine with **calcium** and **iron** from food to form insoluble soaps. These can be harmful in two respects: they can prevent absorption of calcium and iron, causing deficiencies, and can also harden the stools, causing constipation. A fat-free diet is also undesirable because it does not stimulate bile flow and, as a result of this, sediments may form which can promote the development of gallstones.

BIOAVAILABILITY

This term specifies to what extent various micronutrients in food are absorbed and become available to their target tissues or organs after eating. In other words, it is not a matter of what is consumed, but what the body is able to absorb and assimilate from the foods ingested. There is a variety of factors that can influence bioavailability, such as ageing, food processing, reduced digestive secretions, shortage of **enzymes** in the body, and nutrient interaction – in which some nutrients inhibit or increase absorption of other nutrients.

BIOFLAVONOIDS (*Vitamin P*)

Bioflavonoids are complex compounds closely associated with **vitamin C** and found in a wide range of plants, particularly the citrus fruits. All the bioflavonoids enhance the effectiveness of vitamin C, and are recognized as potent **antioxidants**. Together with vitamin C, they strengthen the capillaries and help prevent excessive menstrual bleeding They are also anti-viral and anti-inflammatory, protect from free radicals and inhibit histamine release. Bioflavonoids are therefore indicated in inflammatory and allergic conditions.

As a group, several hundred flavonoids have been identified in fruits, vegetables, nuts, seeds, leaves and flowers. **Onions** and **garlic** provide rich sources of **quercetin**, a bioflavonoid with potent anti-carcinogenic activity which has been shown to inhibit the growth of several types of cancer cells, including breast cancer, ovarian cancer and leukaemia. Quercetin has also been found to be effective in healing wounds, preventing diabetic cataracts and in treating oral herpes.

Cherries, **hawthorn** berries, **blueberries** and other berries are rich in anthocyanidins and proanthocyanidins, the flavonoids that give these berries their dark reddish-blue colour and which are powerful **antioxidants**, preventing free radical damage and helping to maintain healthy collagen and capillaries. **Buckwheat** is rich in the bioflavonoid **rutin,** which is a well-known treatment for haemorrhoids, varicose veins and hypertension. Hesperidin, the predominant flavonoid in citrus fruits, is chemically similar to rutin. Since bioflavonoids strengthen the capillaries, they can assist in the treatment of duodenal ulcers and retinal haemorrhages.

BIOTIN

A water-soluble **B vitamin**, biotin is stable when heated. It is involved in the utilization of **glucose** by increasing insulin action, and can be used in the control of sugar levels in diabetes. It also assists with the utilization of **protein, folic acid** and **vitamin B12**.

Biotin is synthesized in the body by the intestinal bacteria (flora) so that healthy flora are an important factor in the maintenance of correct biotin levels and the prevention of deficiency symptoms. In this respect, **eggs** are best eaten cooked since raw egg white is rich in avidin, a protein that binds biotin and prevents its absorption. Biotin helps to maintain the skin in a healthy condition and alleviate eczema and dermatitis. It also eases muscle aches and is reputed to prevent the hair from greying. Its deficiency symptoms include eczema and dermatitis, lack of **appetite**, fatigue and muscle pains. Biotin is useful in the treatment of hair and scalp conditions. For instance, it is sometimes used in case of hair loss, and a scalp condition in infants known as seborrheic dermatitis appears to improve with biotin supplements. The best natural sources of biotin are **brewer's yeast**, liver, brown **rice**, nuts, egg yolk, **milk** and fruits. The recommended daily dosage is 150–300 mcg. The body's requirement of biotin increases during pregnancy and lactation.

BIRCH, WHITE BIRCH (*BETULA ALBA*)

Also known as the paper birch because its bark separates into
sheets almost like paper, this is a tall, slender tree which grows
wild in northern Europe and North America. Its leaves and
bark are astringent, diuretic and promote perspiration, and
infusions of the leaves are claimed to dissolve kidney stones
and eliminate gravel. Birch can also stimulate kidney functions
and help with the elimination of uric acid. A decoction of
the leaves provides a mild sedative when taken at bedtime.
The decoction is made with one tablespoon of fresh leaves
boiled in half a cup of water. This should be left to steep
for two hours, after which half a teaspoon of bicarbonate of
soda should be added. An infusion can be made with one
tablespoonful of leaves soaked in half a cup of hot water.
Available from larger herbalists.

BIRTH CONTROL PILLS

Birth control pills are known to deplete several important
vitamins in the body such as **B6, folic acid** and **B12**.
Prolonged use of oral **contraceptives** can create typical
deficiency symptoms of these nutrients such as weight
gain, oedema, allergies, anaemia, fatigue, depression and
even loss of sex drive. To prevent such symptoms, long–
term users of the pill would do well to supplement their
diets with these vitamins.

BIRTHWORT (*BETULA ALBA*)

A perennial plant which grows wild in hedges and along fences, both its roots and clustered flower heads can be used for medicinal purposes. The ancient Egyptians used the plant as a remedy for snake bites, and infusions of the roots have traditionally been used to heal ulcers and also to arrest tumours in animals. In addition, infusions of the root and flowers will stimulate perspiration, act as a diuretic, reduce fever and stimulate delayed menstruation. Available from larger health food stores and herbalists. Also incorporated in nutritional formulas.

BISHOP WEED (*AMMI VISNAGA*)

A Middle Eastern herb commonly used in Yemenite and other Arab folk medicine, it contains the glycoside khellin, which has been found to reduce the pain of kidney stones by relieving muscle spasms caused by their pressure. It is also known to alleviate the pain of angina pectoris by dilating the arteries of the heart. Available from larger herbalists.

BITTER MELON (*MOMORDICA CHARANTIA*)

A tropical fruit, also known as balsam pear, bitter melon is a vegetable widely cultivated in Asia, Africa and South America. The fresh juice and the extract of the unripe fruit have been found in various studies to have a **blood sugar** lowering effect. As such, bitter melon is extensively used in folk medicine as a treatment for diabetes.

Bitter melon contains several compounds that have anti-diabetic properties. One of them, charantin, is an efficient sugar-lowering agent composed of mixed steroids. Another active ingredient, momordica, is a polypeptide (**protein**) which reduces blood sugar levels, in much the same way as insulin, when injected into insulin-dependent diabetics. Drinking 50–60 ml of the juice has also shown positive results in clinical trials. Available from larger health food stores and herbalists.

BLACKBERRY (*Rubus villosus*)

A perennial bramble whose sour fruits are rich in **vitamin C** and, especially, anthocyanins, the potent antioxidants of its pigments. Fresh berries are well known for their blood-building properties. Used traditionally as a tonic and to treat anaemia and sore throats, new research shows that blackberries can reduce oestrogen activity and as such are now being tested for use against lung cancer in women.

BLACK COHOSH ROOT (*Cimicifugua racemosa*)

A perennial plant, native to North America, it grows wild from Maine to Missouri, mainly on hillsides. Infusions of the root are astringent, diuretic and anti-spasmodic. Black cohosh was traditionally used by the American Indians to treat female complaints such as menstrual cramps, delayed menstruation and hot flushes of menopause. The root contains 27-deoxyacetin, an active ingredient with oestrogen-like activity. Studies have shown that black cohosh can increase oestrogenic activity and thus alleviate the symptoms of menopause. Recommended for PMT, hot flushes, depression and nervousness. Do not use when pregnant. Available at health food stores.

BLACKCURRANT (*RIBES NIGRUM*)

Best grown in northern regions where the weather is generally cool and wet, blackcurrants were traditionally used, much like blackberries, to prepare delicious drinks, **teas** or home-made syrups. Blackcurrants are extremely rich in **vitamin C**, containing four times as much as the equivalent weight of **oranges**. A 100 g serving can contain up to four times the Recommended Daily Allowance of vitamin C!

The purple-black skins of blackcurants contain anthocyanidins, important antioxidant flavonoids with an anti-inflammatory effect, which explains the practice of sipping hot blackcurrant syrup for sore throats in folk medicine.

Blackcurant seed oil contains essential fatty acids and is one of the richest sources of gamma-linolenic acid (GLA) – in fact it contains about 15 per cent more GLA than **evening primrose oil** – and is sold in capsules under different brand names in health food stores. Applied externally, blackcurrant seed oil can improve skin softness and suppleness.

BLACK NIGHTSHADE (*Solanum nigrum*)

An annual which grows wild on sea cliffs and cultivated land, mainly in England and Wales, although it has been introduced into Scotland and Ireland. It contains several alkaloids, including atropine, solanine and solasodine, a derivative of diosgenin from which plant steroids are made.

Caution: All **nightshades** (see BELLADONNA) are highly poisonous and must be used only under strict medical supervision.

BLOOD CLOTTING

Normal blood clotting is necessary for healing wounds.
Vitamin K promotes blood clotting and is used to prevent or
control internal bleeding and reduce excessive menstrual flow.
However, excessive blood clotting is dangerous and can result
in coronary thrombosis and thrombophlebitis, the main causes
of heart attacks, as well as strokes. The risk of excessive blood
clotting is increased by nutrient deficiencies, alcohol and
excess **arachidonic acid (AA)**, an essential fatty acid prevalent
in **meat**, dairy products, **eggs** and **peanuts**. A **vegetarian
diet** can therefore be beneficial in such cases. A reduction in
blood- clotting can be induced by foods such as **garlic**, **onion**
and oily **fish** (such as **salmon**, mackerel and sardines), and the
use of supplements such as **vitamin E**, **calcium**, **evening
primrose oil**, **omega-3 fatty acids (MaxEPA)**, **lecithin**,
kelp and **octacosanol**, contained in **wheat germ oil**.

BLOOD SUGAR

Since the body burns sugar (**glucose**) for energy, it is
imperative that a consistently adequate blood sugar level is
maintained in order to retain a feeling of well-being – an
ideal blood sugar level is 90–100 mg glucose per 100 cc of
blood. At this level we are energetic and feel good, but
when the level drops to 70 mg, hunger, fatigue and irritability
set in. At levels below this, exhaustion, dizziness, heart
palpitations and nausea are common.

The pancreas is the major sugar regulator, and the body
has a complicated hormonal balancing mechanism which
keeps blood sugar at a fairly constant level. When the level is
too high, the pancreas secretes insulin which converts

glucose to glycogen: when the level is too low, the pancreas secretes glucagon and the adrenal glands secrete adrenalin, two hormones that convert glycogen back to glucose However, if this balancing mechanism gets out of order, it can produce either low blood sugar (hypoglycaemia) or high blood sugar (diabetes). Factors that can affect the blood sugar balance include an excessive use of white sugar, prolonged stress and nutrient deficiencies. Elimination of white sugar from the diet, together with supplements of the B-complex **vitamins**, **chromium** picolinate or GTF chromium, **zinc** and **brewer's yeast** will help to restore and stabilize blood sugar to a more acceptable level.

BLUEBERRIES (*VACCINIUM MYRTILLUS*)

Growing wild in America, Europe and Asia in many varieties, blueberries have been consumed since prehistoric times. But it was only in the twentieth century that they became commercially cultivated. Blueberries are truly a super food. They are the richest of most fruits and vegetables in anthocyanidins, powerful antioxidant **bioflavonoids** contained in their blue, purple and red pigments. With their exceptional antioxidant activity, blueberries were found beneficial in protecting the brain against Alzheimer's disease and the eyes against age-related macular degeneration (AMD). They are now used as an aid in the treatment of urinary tract infections, helping to protect the urethra and bladder from E. coli. Blueberries are also a good source of **vitamin C, fibre, pectin, manganese, vitamin E** and **vitamin B2**. 100 g provide 57 calories, traces of protein and fat, and 14.5 g carbohydrates which consist of 2.4 g fibre and only 9.9 g natural sugars (fructose and glucose).

BLUE GUM TREE SEE EUCALYPTUS

BLUE-GREEN ALGAE (*APHANIZOMENON FLOS-AQUAE*)

Blue-green algae, or AFA, is one of the fastest growing items in the health food market. This unique algae, which is found in Upper Klamath Lake in South Oregon, is considered to be a perfect 'green food' as it contains 60 per cent high-quality **protein**, together with all the essential **amino acids** required for full utilization. It is the richest known source of chlorophyll, which is a blood purifier, is high in **beta** carotene and contains a vast array of **vitamins, minerals** and trace elements, including a high concentration of **vitamin B12**. AFA has been found to have many beneficial effects and regular users report experiencing increased energy and mental alertness, as well as an improvement in conditions such as depression, diabetes, hypoglycaemia, anaemia and Alzheimer's disease. AFA is available from health food shops in capsule, tablet and powder form.

Caution: At the time of publication, some reports have indicated that the supplement may contain toxins linked to paralysis and long-term liver damage.

BONEMEAL

Usually derived from cattle bones, this is a **calcium-phosphorus** supplement that is sold in health food shops in both tablet and powder form. However, since the bonemeal calcium is not chelated, it is best taken with a **protein** meal.

BORAGE OIL

A native of the Mediterranean regions, borage (also called starflower) was brought to Britain by the Romans. The oil of borage is used as a dietary source for gamma-linolenic acid (**GLA**) and, in fact, has been found to provide a more concentrated source of GLA than the more generally used **evening primrose oil** – some batches can be as high in GLA as 20 per cent. A recent study has shown that borage oil can lower hypertension and, as a dietary supplement, has brought about a reduction in high blood pressure within a period of seven weeks. Available from health food stores.

BORON

This trace element was recently found to promote the absorption of **calcium** and **magnesium**. Boron also interacts with **potassium, vitamin D** and **methionine**, and has been found to raise the level of estradiol in women, the most active type of oestrogen. Boron can therefore be beneficial in the menopause, when oestrogen levels drop and calcium absorption is impaired. Boron has also been found to be effective in alleviating symptoms of arthritis, especially juvenile arthritis. Deficiency symptoms of boron include bone demineralisation, brittle bones, arthritis, low oestrogen levels in menopause and reduced growth. The best natural sources of the element are fruits, vegetables and supplements – 3 mg a day provides a normal intake. Although no RDA was established for boron, an upper limit is officially set at 20 mg a day. Available from health food stores on its own or in combination with calcium and multi-mineral formulas.

BRAN

Bran is made up of the fibrous husks that cover grain seeds. It contains 12 per cent polysaccharides (**cellulose, pectin** and lignin) and also **protein**, fat, **vitamins** and **minerals**. Contrary to its common description as 'roughage' food, it is not irritating to the bowels. **Wheat** bran contains 2.5 per cent cellulose (the indigestible part), which compares favourably with **apples** (3.6 per cent) and **grapes** (7 per cent).

However, bran is recommended not so much for its nutritional value, but rather for the ability of its fibre to absorb **water** and give bulk to the faeces. It expands in the colon, stimulating bowel movement and elimination. High-fibre diets speed up waste transit time through the colon, preventing constipation, appendicitis, diverticulosis (pockets in the colon), haemorrhoids and varicose veins, obesity and high blood pressure, cancer of the colon and coronary heart disease. With slow-moving stools, unfriendly bacteria in the colon have time to convert **bile** acids to carcinogens, whereas fast-moving stools facilitate bile excretion, reducing **cholesterol**, hypertension and heart attacks. Wheat bran, oat bran and **rice** bran are among the most popular.

Oat bran has an outstanding soluble fibre content, much more than wheat bran, for example. In many studies, 50–100 g a day of oat bran were found effective in lowering high cholesterol levels, selectively reducing the **LDL** ('bad' cholesterol) level. Oat bran was also found to reduce the need for insulin by 25–50 per cent in adult-onset diabetes. And since oat bran is bulk-forming, it can also contribute to weight loss by curbing the **appetite**. Available from supermarkets and health food stores.

Caution: Consumption of large quantities of raw bran

can result in a deficiency of minerals such as
calcium unless supplements of multi-mineral tablets are
taken.

BRANCHED CHAIN AMINO ACIDS (*BCAA*)

This group contains three essential **amino acids: leucine,
isoleucine** and **valine**. BCAA are essential for muscle
growth and repair, and also help to heal muscle tears,
sprains and tired muscles. They are mostly used, therefore,
by athletes and body builders. BCAA can also help to
strengthen weak muscles after a period of being bedridden
and are good stress relievers. They are available from health
food stores as a food supplement.

BRASSICA

A family of cruciferous vegetables that includes **cabbage,
broccoli, brussels sprouts, cauliflower** and **kale**. They
are rich in **vitamins** and **minerals**, particularly **sulphur**,
the 'beauty mineral' which produces collagen and boosts
the immune system against germs and viruses. They also
contain compounds with anti-cancer properties, such as
dithiolthiones and indoles which protect against breast and
colon cancer. This family of vegetables also has a beneficial
effect on the liver.

BREAST FEEDING SEE BABIES, FOOD

BREWER'S YEAST

A unicellular micro-organism, brewer's yeast was originally a by-product of the brewing industry that grew on **hops**, grain or malt, and which had to be debittered. Now, due to is high nutritional value, brewer's yeast is mainly produced as a supplement. The best types are those graded 'primary'. These are usually grown on **molasses** or sugar beets and are pleasant-tasting.

Brewer's yeast is a well-balanced food, containing excellent concentrations of **B-complex vitamins**, including even **vitamin B12** in some cases. It is up to 45 per cent complete **protein**, containing 17 **amino acids**, including all the essential ones, and is a rich source of DNA and RNA, which together form 12 per cent of dried yeast. It also contains an abundance of **minerals** and trace elements. For example, it is high in **iron** and **copper**, making it helpful in the treatment of anaemia. In addition, it contains high amounts of **chromium** and **glucose tolerance factor (GTF)** which benefits diabetics and hypoglycaemics. It also contains **selenium** – in fact, some yeasts are actually grown on selenium, making them 'selenium-rich yeast'. This selenium, in particular, is easily absorbed. Initially, only small amounts of brewer's yeast should be taken on a daily basis; then, as the body adapts to it, the amounts can gradually be increased. It is available from health food shops in tablet, flake or powder form.

Caution: Brewer's yeast is contra-indicated in cases of candida (thrush).

BROCCOLI (*BRASSICA OLERACEA*)

A member of the **Brassica** family, broccoli is a green vegetable that can be eaten either raw or cooked. Broccoli is exceptionally nutritious, containing an abundance of **sulphur, iron** and chlorophyll, which purifies the blood; it is also rich in **vitamins A, B-complex** and especially **C**. In fact, it contains more **vitamin C** than **oranges** – one cup provides as much as 70 mg of vitamin C.

Known for its great cancer-combating ability, broccoli was found to contain sulphoraphane, a sulphur-based compound, which helps to kill cancer-causing substances in food. When sulphoraphane is released in the gut, it steps up production of powerful enzymes that destroy carcinogenic substances such as those found in heavily barbecued meat. Another naturally occurring compound found in broccoli – I3C – was found in a US study to increase DNA repair proteins, thus preventing genetic information damage and lowering the risk of developing cancer. And a recent British study with people who had precancerous prostate cells confirmed that a diet rich in broccoli produced changes in gene activity that stopped or slowed down cancer cell growth. **Caution**: Broccoli should be avoided in cases of thyroid deficiency.

BROMELAIN

A **protein**-splitting enzyme present in pineapple, which has traditionally been used in the Caribbean regions as **meat** tenderizer. This is why pineapple can combine well with meat dishes. As a supplemental digestive aid, bromelain is available in health food shops in tablet and capsule form.

BRUSSELS SPROUTS (*BRASSICA OLERACEA*)

A member of the **Brassica** family of vegetables, Brussels sprouts are similar to **cabbage** in fl vour and nutrient content and provide an excellent source of **vitamins C, B1** and **beta carotene**. Similarly, they are also rich in **potassium**, **calcium** and **sulphur** but, unlike **cabbage** and **broccoli**, which can be enjoyed both raw and cooked, Brussels sprouts are palatable only as a cooked vegetable.

BUCHU (*BOROSMA BETULINA*)

A small shrub native to South Africa, where its leaves are dried and used as a **tea** that is drunk as a tonic. It is also exported to Britain and the USA, where it is recognized as an excellent herb tea for those who suffer from cystic, urinary gravel and other urinary problems. Available from health food stores.

BUCKWHEAT, KASHA

Buckwheat is an **alkali-forming** grain which, when roasted, is known as 'kasha'. As a very rich source of **rutin**, buckwheat helps strengthen capillaries, inhibit inner bleeding, prevent and treat haemorrhoids and varicose veins, and helps lower high blood pressure. It is also rich in **fibre** and silica, which strengthens the intestines and helps treat chronic diarrhoea. Buckwheat contains chiro-inositol, which increases sensitivity to insulin, and a new Canadian study found that it can be beneficial to patients with type 2 diabetes Sprouted buckwheat is rich in chlorophyll, **vitamins** and **enzymes**. Available at supermarkets and health food stores.

BURDOCK (*Arctium lappa*)

A small biennial plant which grows wild in North America and Europe, its leaves, roots and seeds all have nutritional and medicinal uses. It is a diuretic and blood cleanser, promotes perspiration and stimulates digestion. In addition, burdock also has anti-fungal, anti-bacterial and anti-tumour factors. As such it is used to treat chronic skin disorders like eczema and help prevent cancerous growths.

Burdock also contains the polysaccharide inulin, which is known to reduce inflammation and, as an anti-bacterial, it can help with the treatment of staph infections.

The fresh plant is used in macrobiotic cooking. For infusions and decoctions, the fresh root can be grated to a juice, or used dried. It is available from health food stores in capsule form. It is also incorporated in nutritional formulas and is available as a dried herb from herbalists.

BUTCHER'S BROOM (*Ruscus aculeatus*)

An evergreen shrub of the lily family, the rhizome of the plant has medicinal properties as it contains active alkaloids that have many physiological effects. For instance, they are anti-inflammatory and can constrict blood vessels. The plant was traditionally used in treating vein disorders, both internally and externally, such as haemorrhoids and varicose veins. In addition, infusions made from the rhizome are recognized as a good herbal drink for jaundice, oedema and gout.

Capsules are available from health food stores. It is also incorporated in nutritional formulas and is available as a dried herb from herbalists.

BUTTER, BUTYRIC ACID

Produced by churning pasteurized cream, butter consists mainly of saturated fat with some water and a scant amount of **protein** (casein), unsaturated fatty acids, lactose and minerals. Although, like any saturated fat it contains **cholesterol**, it is still less harmful than standard **margarine**. For instance, butter contains from 4–6 per cent essential fatty acids, which help to prevent heart attacks, while margarine contains only 2–5 per cent. While butter can only have salt as one added ingredient, margarines have colourings, emulsifiers, preservatives and synthetic vitamins added to them. Nutritionists are now increasingly realizing that it is the saturated fats in foods like margarine, not dietary cholesterol, that raise blood cholesterol levels.

Butter is a rich source of easily absorbed **vitamin A** and butyric acid, a short-chain fatty acid needed for cell health and repair, especially of the colon. It is also a natural source of vitamins **E, K** and **D**. Among its trace minerals, it contains **selenium**, an important cancer-protecting element which is commonly deficient in many people.

As with other **fats**, when heated above certain temperatures, butter oxidises and decomposes, producing irritating substances in the digestive tract. For frying purposes, it is important to note that the fatty acids in butter decompose at 226°F (108°C). It is best to adjust frying temperatures accordingly, and never re-fry previously heated butter.

C

CABBAGE (*BRASSICA OLERACEA*)

One of the **Brassica** family, cabbage provides a rich source of **vitamin C** – in fact, the vitamin C content of cabbage is greater than that of **oranges**. It also contains a large number of **minerals**, including **iodine**, **sulphur**, **calcium**, **magnesium** and **potassium**. The outer leaves contain more **vitamin E** and calcium than the inner leaves. If prepared as **sauerkraut**, it makes an excellent food for strengthening the intestines and promoting a healthy flora.

Cabbage is recommended in natural medicine practice for improving digestion, treating constipation, preventing the common cold and alleviating depression. It also contains a factor called **vitamin U**, which is a remedy for ulcers, and raw cabbage juice has been reported to assist in the cure of both peptic and duodenal ulcers. The recommended method is to drink half a cup of freshly made cabbage juice two or three times a day between meals, on an empty stomach.

Many of the healing properties of cabbage as a blood purifier are due to its high sulphur content. Grated cabbage can also be made into a poultice to be applied externally in the treatment of wounds, varicose veins and leg ulcers.

CADMIUM

Cadmium is a highly toxic element – as little as one-half to one ppm in **water** can be toxic – and, once in the body, cadmium displaces **zinc** and accumulates in the kidneys, liver and blood vessels, probably for life.

Cadmium occurs naturally in zinc ores, but is also a typical environmental pollutant and, since it is present in car exhaust fumes, it pollutes the air of all major cities. It is also found in cigarette smoke – a 20-pack of cigarettes contains 20 mg of cadmium, half of which is absorbed during smoking. Nickel-cadmium battery plants are well- known sources of pollution, as are incinerators of discarded cars, and zinc- and **copper**-smelting plants. Cadmium is also contained in phosphate fertilizers, via which it can contaminate vegetation. Cadmium is also found in drinking **water** from corroded pipes, especially soft water which increases corrosion.

Cadmium is one of the major contributors to high blood pressure, atherosclerosis, strokes and heart attacks. Emphysema patients have been found to have more cadmium in their kidneys and liver than healthy people – cigarette smoking, in particular, has been associated with emphysema because of the cadmium content of cigarette smoke.

Nutritional protection from the toxic effects of cadmium can be provided by zinc, which replaces cadmium, and by large doses of **vitamin C**.

CAFFEINE, COFFEE

Caffeine is the most prevalent stimulant in western society since it is present in coffee, **tea**, cocoa, **chocolate** and colas, as well as in many over-the-counter stimulants and drugs such as analgesics. It has been estimated that the average daily caffeine consumption per person is 150–225 mg, 75 per cent of which comes from coffee. A cup of coffee contains 50–150 mg of caffeine, while a cup of **tea** contains about 50 mg and a 340 g can of cola contains about 35 mg.

However, caffeine consumption in heavy coffee drinkers is far higher – in some cases this can be anything up to 7,500 mg a day! The excessive and prolonged intake of coffee can cause 'caffeinism' symptoms such as anxiety, nervousness, insomnia, depression, constipation, frequent urination, duodenal ulcers, high **cholesterol**, hypertension and heart disease; it is also believed to be involved in a proneness to breast lumps, while coffee drinking during pregnancy is thought to increase the risk of miscarriage.

People who are sensitive to caffeinism can exhibit some of these symptoms from as few as two cups of coffee a day.

In addition, caffeine inhibits absorption of **iron**, promoting anaemia, it can create deficiencies of **inositol, calcium** and **magnesium** as it interferes with their absorption, and, since it raises the cholesterol level, it can increase susceptibility to heart attack. Coffee is not recommended for people with gout or kidney stones. Caffeine contains purines, which break-down in the body to uric acid, promoting the formation of kidney stones and gouty crystals.

However, a new Harvard study suggests that two to three cups of coffee a day can lower the risk of developing gallstones. Externally, coffee can be used in anemas and in poultices to heal bruises.

CALCIUM

Calcium is the most abundant mineral in the human body, with almost all of it – 99 per cent – found in the bones and the teeth, helping to build bone mass and preventing osteoporosis (bone loss). However, the remaining 1 per cent, which is in blood, is of paramount importance to the body as it normalizes nerve and muscle function, regulates heart-beat, enables **blood clotting**, helps to maintain a proper acid-alkaline balance, induces sleep and promotes skin health.

Unfortunately, absorption of calcium in the body is very inefficient and there are a number of factors needed for its proper absorption, including stomach acid (HCl), **vitamins A, C** and **D, magnesium** and **protein**. In addition, regular **exercise** will promote calcium deposition in bones, while a sedentary lifestyle depletes it, causing porous bones. Pregnant and menopausal women, especially, are very vulnerable to calcium deficiencies and bone loss unless

they take calcium supplements. Older men can also be prone to calcium deficiency and also people with digestive disorders, such as ulcers or Crohn's disease, because of the accompanying reduction in stomach secretions. Coffee, alcohol, soft drinks, diuretics, **antacids** and excess protein can all deplete calcium levels.

Deficiency symptoms include brittle bones, tooth decay, nervousness, muscle aches, leg cramps, excessive menstrual flow and impaired growth. A high supplement of calcium (1–2 g per day) not only helps to reverse osteoporosis, but also treats conditions such as high **cholesterol** levels and hypertension. Among the best natural sources are dairy products, **sesame seeds**, soya beans, **peanuts**, green vegetables, **sunflower seeds**, bone-marrow soups and calcium tablets. Calcium citrate is considered to be the most efficiently absorbed form of calcium, and has the least risk of causing kidney stones.

The normal Recommended Daily Allowance of calcium for adults is 800 mg, while the recommended daily dosage for pregnant and lactating women is 1,200 mg. However, many experts recommend higher doses of up to 1,5000 mg per day.

CALCIUM ASCORBATE

This is the acid-free form of **vitamin C** in which calcium is used to buffer the acidity of vitamin C. It is usually recommended for people who suffer from stomach overacidity, those prone to ulcers and people with frequent heartburn.

CALENDULA (*CALENDULA OFFICINALIS*)

Commonly known as marigold, calendula is an annual garden plant. An infusion of the flowers, or the fresh juice, can be used for digestive tract problems such as stomach cramps, gastritis, ulcers, colitis and diarrhoea. It has a soothing effect and can also be used for boils, bruises and wounds.

Calendula has been traditionally used for its beneficial effects on skin problems. Calendula extracts penetrate the skin tissue, relax the skin and reduce swellings. Special calendula extracts are claimed to tighten the skin and improve the complexion. Available in health food stores in dried form and creams.

CALORIE

A calorie is a unit of energy that represents the amount of heat required to raise the temperature of 1 g of **water** by 34°F (1°C). In terms of human nutrition, calories are a measurement of the energy produced when food is metabolized by the body. Thus, calorific values denote the amount of heat energy yielded by different foods, and are usually expressed on food labels as Kcal (kilo calorie) units.

Different types of foods supply different amounts of

calories – for instance, **proteins** and **carbohydrates** provide 4 Kcal per g each, while **fats** provide 9 Kcal per g – and the calories received from food are 'burned' in the course of our daily activities. Thus, in a perfect situation, the amount of calories consumed from food should equal the amount of calories spent. In such cases, the energy flow is balanced. However, when more calories are eaten than spent, the excess calories are stored as fat and the result is weight gain. Conversely, eating fewer calories than the body requires will result in weight loss. So 0.4 kg of body fat equals 3,500 calories, but the daily calorie requirement for each individual varies greatly according to age, sex, body type, genetic predisposition and lifestyle.

However, not all calories are created equal. Slimmers should remember that sugar calories are more fattening than **protein** or complex carbohydrate calories.

CALORIE-RESTRICTED DIETS

Calorie-restricted diets with proper supplementation have found to extend the life span of laboratory animals. Young animals restricted to 60 per cent of their normal food intake lived up to 50 per cent longer than animals with no food limits. In addition, the animals that ate less were much healthier and looked youthful into their old age. The anti-ageing effects of calorie restriction were discovered as early as 1934, but until recently it was not known how this works. However, research has now shown that food restriction retards the ageing of the pineal gland. This is the gland that produces **melatonin**, a hormone that greatly influences our health and well-being, and production of which decreases with age. Studies done by life insurance companies have shown that, statistically, overweight people have the shortest life span while those whose weight is just below the average have the longest life span.

CAMOMILE (*MATRICARIA CHAMOMILLA*)

An annual plant, native to Mediterranean countries, it is now widely cultivated in other regions such as the British Isles. The herb has long been used for its calming effect and has also been found to be beneficial in the t eatment of indigestion, colic, spasms, stomach cramps and insomnia. Camomile has antiseptic properties and can be used to alleviate inflammation of the digest ve tract. It also contains apigenin, a chemical which was found to inhibit the spreading rate of breast cancer cells in studies at the Ohio State University. In addition, it is used in mouthwashes and gargles, as well as in sitz-baths to relieve haemorrhoids. The dried fl wers are very popular as a herb tea.

CANOLA OIL

This is produced from the canola variety of rapeseed which has a high content of a monounsaturated fat, oleic acid. Canola oil is often recommended because of its low saturated fat content (6 per cent), its **omega-3 fatty acids** (10 per cent) and especially for its monounsaturates (60 percent), which make it safer and healthier than most other vegetable oils. The oil is used by food processing companies to make cooking oil and products such as **margarine** and salad dressings.

CAPRYLIC ACID

A naturally occurring fatty acid commercially derived from **coconut** oil. Caprylic acid has been found to have antifungal properties and is used to treat candida albicans (thrush). It is absorbed in the intestines, and the tablets should be enteric-coated, or time-release, to protect them during their passage through the stomach, until they reach the intestines. Available from health food stores.

CARAWAY (*CARUM CARVI*)

A biennial cultivated herb, its seed are commonly used for flavouring foods, especially bread. Caraway can stimulate the **appetite**, relieve flatulence and improve digestion. It can also promote the onset of menstruation and alleviate uterine cramps. To prepare an infusion, use one teaspoon of crushed seeds boiled in half a cup of **water**. Available from supermarkets or health food stores.

CARBOHYDRATES

As a group of organic chemical compounds, carbohydrates are classified as macronutrients. Carbohydrates molecules are made up of carbon, hydrogen and oxygen and are the body's chief source of energy. As such they are known as 'energy food'. Carbohydrates are supplied mainly from plant foods, such as **grains**, pulses, fruits and vegetables. Sugar is 100 per cent carbohydrate, cornflakes are 85 per cent, **rice** 79, flour 73, pasta 70, **oats** 61, bread 47, potato 20, **banana** 21 and **apple** 12 per cent.

Carbohydrates come in several varieties and types:

monosaccharides, or simple sugars, which include **glucose, fructose** and galactose, found in fruits and **honey**; disaccharides, the more complex sugars, which include sucrose (in cane and **beet** sugar), **lactose** (in **milk**) and maltose (in malted **barley**); and finally, polysaccharides, or complex carbohydrates, which include starch, **cellulose** (fibre) and glycogen.

All carbohydrates except cellulose are ultimately converted in the body to glucose. This is the sole usable form of energy, and the body depends on a continuous supply of it for all its activities, mental and physical.

Carbohydrates yield 4 **calories** per g. The most widely used carbohydrate is sucrose, or refined sugar. Calories derived from sugar through sweetened foods and drinks have been termed 'empty calories', because these foods lack the essential **vitamins, minerals** and other nutrients that accompany whole natural fruits in nature, such as the sugar cane and beets from which they are derived. Excess consumption of refined sugar can have many detrimental effects, from tooth decay, obesity and fatigue to high **cholesterol** levels, hypoglycaemia and diabetes. Sugar is also a stressing food.

CARDAMOM (*ELETTARIA CARDAMOMUM*)

A perennial plant that grows wild in India, it is now cultivated in other tropical areas of the world. The seeds of the plant, which are enclosed in fruity pods, have both medicinal and culinary uses. Cardamom is known as a carminative, relieving flatulence, stimulating the stomach and aiding digestion. However, it is mainly used as a cooking spice or for flavouring drinks and medicines. In Arab countries it is commonly added to coffee. Widely available.

CARNITINE, L-CARNITINE

A non-essential amino acid that plays a part in the utilization of **fats** in the body, it also helps to transport fatty acids to the mitochondria, the tiny power plants in the cells that convert fat to energy. Thus, by reducing triglyceride levels, supplemental carnitine can help to reduce angina pectoris attacks and provide protection from heart failure. Carnitine also inhibits the development of fatty liver disease induced by alcohol, and assists with weight loss, fighting fatigue and the release of more energy.

Carnitine is supplied mostly from animal food (**meat** and dairy) but is also manufactured by the body (in the liver and kidneys) from the **amino acids lysine** and **methionine**. Carnitine deficiencies can occur in people on low-**protein** diets or when **vitamins B** and **C** and **iron** are in short supply. Carnitine supplements are widely available in health food shops and pharmacies. People likely to benefit most from carnitine supplements include strict **vegetarians** and **vegans**, slimmers on crash diets, body builders, senior citizens and people with heart or kidney disease.

CAROB (*CERATONIA SILIQUA*)

Also called locust bean, carob has been known since biblical times as St John's bread. The carob is an evergreen tree, native to Mediterranean countries, which is found both wild and cultivated. The carob produces long pods containing both gum and seeds, both of which have culinary and medicinal uses.

The gum, which has a flavour similar to cocoa, is rich in natural sugars such as galactomannan, **calcium** and **minerals**. Carob powder, produced from the dried gum, is now increasingly used commercially in confectionery and biscuits as a **chocolate** substitute for people allergic to chocolate. The food industry also uses carob as an emulsifier and stabiliser (E410) in many foods, such as ice creams, soups and salad dressings. Carob powder is available in health food stores as a cocoa substitute for home baking purposes.

CAROTENOIDS

This is the common name for several hundred plant pigments which are powerful **antioxidants**. Found in fruits such as cantaloupe, **papaya** and **pumpkin** and vegetables such as **carrots, tomatoes** and red **grapes**, carotenoids absorb the dangerous sun rays that produce free radicals. These free radicals are extremely harmful, not only to plants but also to humans where they can cause the degenerative diseases of ageing such as heart disease, cancer and arthritis. Thus, the inclusion in the diet of plenty of fresh fruit and vegetables containing carotenoids can help to provide protection from the damaging effects of free radicals. Some carotenoids, such as alpha, beta and gamma carotenes, are also **vitamin A** precursors. Non-provitamin A dietary carotenoids include **lycopene**, lutein and zeaxanthin. There are indications that lycopene, found mainly in tomatoes, may help to lower the risk of prostate cancer, while alpha carotene, found in carrots, may provide protection from other forms of cancer. Lutein and zeaxanthin found in green vegetables such as **peppers, spinach**, collards green and **kale**, were found to prevent age-related macular degeneration of the eye (AMD) which can lead to loss of central vision in people over 50. Carotenoids are also available in capsules as nutritional supplements, particularly in antioxidant formulas.

CARRAGEENAN

Carrageenan is a jellying compound extracted from red **seaweeds** (algae). Traditionally, the Irish extracted it from Irish moss (*Chondrus crispus*) and used it as a food and a remedy for respiratory diseases. Commercially, carrageenan was not produced until the Second World War, when an alternative to the Japanese **agar** (E406) was needed.

Carrageenan is composed of several hydrocolloids, rather than a single substance. It consists of varying amounts of **calcium, magnesium**, ammonium, **potassium** and **sodium** salts of sulphate esters of galactose and 3,6-anhydrogalactose copolymers. The carrageenan used in food has a high molecular weight and comprises all the long chain molecules of the copolymers. This is termed 'food grade carrageenan'. Degraded carrageenan has a low molecular weight with no jellying properties.

Carrageenan comes in the form of a dried, translucent mucilage that swells in cold water, dissolving partially to make a jelly. It is used (in low concentrations of up to 1 per cent) in the food industry as a stabilizing, thickening, suspending and jellying agent. For example, it is extensively used as a stabilizer of **milk proteins** in such products as ice cream, milk shakes and milk **chocolate** (E407).

Degraded carrageenan was found to cause ulcerative colitis and tumours in animals. This is why use was forbidden by EEC statutory regulations, which has led to public confusion about the safety of carrageenan. However, although carrageenan undergoes some degradation in the acid environment of the stomach, small amounts do not appear to cause any harm; it is only in large amounts that it is suspected of being a health hazard.

CARROT (*Daucus carota*)

A common root vegetable, it is one of the richest sources of **beta carotene**, a **vitamin A** precursor. Carrots are also an excellent source of **vitamins B1** and **B2** and of the **minerals potassium, sodium** and **silicon**. Carrots have been reported to help night vision, inhibit cataracts, treat indigestion and protect against cancer. They are also thought to be useful in treating infections of the lung, digestive system and urinary tract. Regular inclusion in the diet of raw or cooked carrots can improve skin appearance and **calcium** absorption, while cooked carrots can benefit people with weak digestion. Carrot juice, while pleasant on its own, also provides a good basis for the addition of other less palatable juices such as **celery** or **beet**.

    Caution: It is recommended that the intake of carrot juice should be limited to no more than four cups a day since over-consumption can cause yellowing of the skin, a condition known as xanthosis.

CARTILAGE, SHARK AND BOVINE

Sharks have long been known for their high resistance to disease and wound healing ability. Unlike other vertebrates, the shark's skeleton in composed of a special cartilage, and it is to this that its healing properties are attributed.

    The cartilage of the shark has been found to have strong anti-cancer and anti-inflammatory effects which, when used on humans, can help to restore flexibility to arthritic joints and inhibit the growth of malignant tumours. Recently, attention has also been focused on bovine cartilage which appears to have similar properties. Most of the studies done have confirmed its efficacy and, in fact, suggest that much lower doses of bovine than shark cartilage are required to be effective, making its use more practical. Available from health food stores.

CASCARA SAGRADA (*RHAMNUS PURSHIANA OR R. CATHARTICUS*)

A small tree or shrub that is native to North America, its Spanish name means 'sacred bark', and it is the bark of the tree that has traditionally been used as a herbal laxative. In some countries it is dispensed as a prescription herb, and its active ingredients include certain glycosides (anthraquinones) and bitter principles which act on the bowels, increasing their movement and promoting evacuation. Cascara is generally considered safe. However, when used in excessive dosages or over prolonged periods of time, it can cause toxic reactions. Cascara is available in several forms, such as the dried herb and as an extract, and it is increasingly used in laxative formulas sold in health food shops.

CASHEW NUT (*ANACARDIUM OCCIDENTALE*)

A bean-shaped nut that grows on tropical evergreen trees native to Central America, the cashew which has become a popular snack all over the world, is very nutritious. It is rich in **protein** (18 per cent), a variety of minerals (especially copper, iron, magnesium and zinc), several B vitamins and vitamin E. Out of a total of 30 per cent carbohydrate, three per cent is fibre and 100 grams provide 553 calories. Their high fat content of 43 per cent is "heart friendly". It is made up mostly of monounsaturated fatty acids (like oleic and palmitoleic) which help reduce LDL ("bad") cholesterol, and help prevent coronary heart disease and strokes. Cashews are also marketed as "cashew butter". Due to their high fat content, cashews are preferably eaten raw rather than roasted.

CAT'S CLAW (*UNCARIA TOMENTOSA*)

A thorny vine native to the Amazon rainforest, it has been hailed in recent years as an immune system booster and has been found to be beneficial in the treatment of cancer and AIDS. The herb is currently being researched, with studies checking its possible benefits in the treatment of arthritis, allergies, ulcers and acne. One study found that it may help relieve the knee pain of osteoarthritis without significant side effects. Increasingly sought after in health food shops, where it is sold as a tea and as capsules.

CATNIP (*NEPETA CATARIA*)

Also known as catmint, this is an aromatic perennial herb of the mint family. Its leaves can be used to make an effective infusion for an upset stomach, colic and flatulence. It can also be used in enemas. Available from health food stores, incorporated in nutritional formulas, and from herbalists.

CAULIFLOWER (*Brassica oleracea*)

A very nutritious vegetable of the **Brassica** family, it is rich in **vitamins C, B1** and **B2** and is a good source of **calcium, magnesium, phosphorus, potassium** and **sulphur**. It is usually cooked but can be eaten raw or is pickled. It should be stored in the refrigerator, and when selecting cauliflower look for fresh compact heads, with no discoloration; if the buds are spread out or spotted, this means that the cauliflower is old or has been exposed too long to the sun. Anyone with a sensitive digestion may find that the raw vegetable causes flatulence or bloating and, in such cases, it is advisable to slightly cook or sauté the cauliflower.

CAYENNE PEPPER (*Capsicum frutescens*)

Originally a perennial plant native to the tropical regions of Central America, it is now cultivated elsewhere as an annual. The fruits, or hot **peppers**, commonly known as chillis, contain capsaicin, a stimulant that helps to control pain and dissolve blood clots. Chillis can stimulate the **appetite** and digestion, release phlegm and increase sweating and resistance to colds. In moderation, powdered chillis can help heal stomach and duodenal ulcers, promoting tissue growth through the release of histamine. Cayenne pepper is also effective in the treatment of ailments as diverse as arthritis, asthma, diabetes, high blood pressure, kidney infections, sinusitis and other respiratory problems, as well as reputedly providing a remedy for hangovers.

CELERY (*APIUM GRAVEOLENS VAR. DULCE*)

A popular vegetable related to **carrots** and **parsley**, it
probably originated in the Mediterranean regions. The
vegetable is available all–year round and provides a good
source of **vitamins A, B1** and **B2**, as well as the
minerals calcium, phosphorus and **silicon**. Especially
rich in **potassium** and **sodium**, four fresh stalks of celery
provide 341 mg potassium and 126 mg sodium, and their
juice makes a great electrolyte replacement drink.
Coumarin compounds in the celery appear to be useful in
toning the heart and blood vessels. These compounds can
also be useful in cases of migraine. One of them, 3–n–butyl
phthalide, was found to significantly lower blood pressure.
The stalks of the plant, which are rich in **iron,
magnesium** and carotene, are usually eaten raw in salads
or with dips, or are used in soups and as a garnish for
other foods. They are high in roughage and, when eaten
between meals, can help with **appetite** control. On the
other hand, the leaves are thought to stimulate the appetite,
and also increase urination and bring on menstruation. Celery
juice has been used to alleviate oedema, treat rheumatism and
clear skin problems and, combined with a little **lemon** juice,
it can help to prevent a cold developing. Both the stalks and
roots are used to treat hypertension,
and the seeds are used as a sedative and to relieve
flatulence. A decoction of the seeds can be used as a
remedy for rheumatism and bronchitis, and for calming
frayed nerves. Dried ground celery is sold as a **salt**
substitute for low **sodium** diets.

CELLULOSE

As a fibrous from of complex carbohydrates, cellulose is a component of plant cell walls that is indigestible and insoluble in **water**. However, it has the ability to bind with water and increase stool mass and weight, promoting bowel movement and elimination. Moreover, it also speeds up stool transit time, i.e. the time needed for food to travel from mouth to anus. Thus, it helps to prevent severe colon conditions such as constipation, diverticulitis and cancer of the colon. Small parts of cellulose ferment and degrade in the colon, and this degradation produces **short chain fatty acids** which are important for the energy metabolism of the colon. A major source of cellulose is **wheat bran.**

CENTAURY (*CENTAURIUM ERYTHRAEA*)

This small annual herb grows wild on chalk downs and sandy soils throughout Europe. The small pink or white flowers are taken as an infusion before meals to stimulate **appetite** and aid digestion by encouraging the liver to secrete **bile**. It can also act as a blood purifier and help to reduce fever. Applied externally, centaury is reputed to repel fleas and lice. Available from larger health food stores and herbalists.

CETYL MYRISTOLEATE (CM)

Discovered in the 1960s, CM has recently received much publicity due to its beneficial effect in treating various types of arthritis. Cetyl myristoleate is an ester of a fatty acid which occurs in very small amounts in all **fats** and oils. It is made by taking the fatty acid myristoleic acid,

obtained from the palmitic acid in **coconut** and palm
oils, and combining it with a long chain alcohol molecule.
Commercially, CM is known as a super lubricant. At room
temperature it is a waxy, buttery substance.

CM was found to be beneficial in several ways for both
osteoarthritis and rheumatic arthritis. It lubricates not only the
inflamed joints, but also the entire body, softening the tissues,
making them more pliable and enabling muscles to glide
more smoothly over each other and over bursas and bones.
And as a good fatty acid, CM also helps reduce inflammations.
Moreover, CM appears to modulate the immune system, which
may explain its beneficial effect in treating such auto-immune
diseases as rheumatoid arthritis, multiple sclerosis and lupus
erythematosus. Several studies showed that CM can be effective
in treating up to 87 per cent of various forms of arthritis. CM
is available as a food supplement, usually sold under the trade
name of CELADRIN, and can be taken with **glucosamine
sulphate**, hydrolyzed **cartilage** and M.S.M. for increased effect.

CHERRY (*PRUNUS*)

The fruit of an attractive tree, native to Europe and Western
Asia, and extensively grown in America in sour and sweet
varieties, cherries were traditionally used in folk medicine
as an effective treatment for arthritis, gout and rheumatism.
Cherries are rich sources of flavonoids such as anthocyanidins
and proanthocyanidins which give the fruits their deep red-
blue colour. These flavonoids are potent **antioxidants** which
make them useful in treating a variety of inflammations by
inhibiting histamine release. They protect collagen from free
radical damage, help prevent wrinkles and also reduce uric
acid levels, thus benefiting gout. 225g of the fresh fruit a

day constitutes a treatment for lowering uric acid levels and preventing attacks of gout.

CHESTNUTS (*Castanea crenata*)

Traditionally roasted and consumed during winter months, chestnuts are considerably higher in carbohydrates and much lower in protein and fat than other nuts. Chestnuts contain four times as much carbohydrates, one third of the protein and one fifteenth of the at, but only half of the calories, compared to other nuts. Chestnuts are a good source of potassium, magnesium, iron and manganese, although in lower amounts of other nuts. Due to their low fat content, chestnuts store rather well.

CHIA SEEDS (*Salvia Hispanica*)

Hailed in recent years as a super food, Chia was traditionally cultivated in South America by the Aztecs as an important food crop. Modern studies showed that Chia seeds are indeed loaded with a vast array of essential nutrients. High in B vitamins, especially **thiamine (B1)** and **niacin (B3)**, they are also a rich source of minerals such as **calcium, magnesium, iron, manganese, phosphorus** and **zinc**. A serving of 28 g contains 137 calories and provides: Protein 4g, carbohydrates 12g (of which 11g are fibre), fat 9g (of which 6.7g are polyunsaturated, 5g are **omega-3**). Due to their high fibre content, Chia seeds absorb 10 times their weight in water. They form a jellylike mass in the gut, contributing to a feeling of fullness, thus helping to lose weight. The seeds can be added to other foods such as soups, porridges, puddings, yogurt or smoothies. While preliminary research indicated that Chia seeds provide potential health benefits, definitive therapeutic results were sparse and inconclusive. Nevertheless, the seeds are considered to be useful in various conditions such as diabetes, constipation, anaemia, high blood pressure, brittle bones, fatigue and overweight.

CHICKPEA (*Cicer arietinum*)

Also called the garbanzo bean, this is a versatile bean which is recently gaining popularity in dishes like hummus, falafel, curries and stews. Increasingly grown in subtropical areas like Turkey, Mexico and India, chickpeas are an excellent source of protein, especially when combined with grains like rice, which raises their protein availability. Like other beans, chickpeas are rich in both soluble and insoluble **dietary fibre**, which helps lower cholesterol levels, increase stool bulk and prevent constipation. Having a low **Glycaemic Index**, they can benefit dietes. Chickpeas are also a rich source of folic acid and of minerals like **iron, manganese, zinc** and **molybdenum**.

CHICORY (*Cichorium intybus*)

A perennial plant that is cultivated in North America and Europe, mainly for its edible leaves and roots, it was popular with both the Ancient Egyptians and Greeks for its culinary and medicinal properties. Infusions or decoctions of the root or fl wers can stimulate the **appetite**, aid digestion, promote **bile** secretion and help to relieve the pain and discomfort caused by gallstones. Dried ground chicory is used as a coffee substitute, either on its own or, combined with cereals, in cereal coffees. Available from supermarkets, grocers and health food stores.

CHILLI see CAYENNE PEPPER

CHLORELLA

A green freshwater algae, chlorella is now being marketed in health food shops as a food supplement. About 60 per cent of chlorella is in the form of high-quality **protein**, about 20 per cent consists of carbohydrates and 10 per cent is fat. It contains more than 20 different **vitamins** and **minerals**, is a rich source of **beta carotene** and contains more **vitamin B12** than beef liver. Chlorella contains appreciable amounts of **iron, iodine, zinc** and **cobalt**. It is also one of the richest sources of chlorophyll and DNA.

Due to its richness in essential nutrients, many beneficial effects have been attributed to chlorella. It is reputed to stimulate the immune system and help to reduce the risk of some cancers; it has also been used to treat anaemia, fatigue, hypertension, diabetes and constipation. In addition, its high chlorophyll content makes chlorella a useful blood purifier.

CHLOROPHYLL

Chlorophyll is the green pigment in plants that enables photosynthesis, i.e. it enables sunshine to combine carbon dioxide with **water**, creating **carbohydrates** and oxygen. By utilizing light, chlorophyll is a primary source of plant energy. Its chemical structure is similar to haemoglobin (the red blood pigment that carries oxygen), which is why it is used in the treatment of certain anaemias.

It can promote growth, metabolism and respiration and has the ability to stimulate tissue growth and wound healing. Chlorophyll cream has been used to treat skin ulcers and when injected it can help to reduce **cholesterol** levels. It is also known as a blood purifier, detoxifier and deodorizer.

Chlorophyll has many commercial and therapeutic applications. For instance, it is widely used in colouring food and cosmetics (E140), and a common brand of breath-refreshing chewing gum contains chlorophyll.

CHOCOLATE

A delicious recreational food, chocolate is one of the yummy 'sins' of civilization. Chocolate is made from the beans of the cocoa tree (*Theobroma cacao*), a native of Mexico since the time of the Aztecs who named it 'chocolatl', and who also used its beans as currency. The beans are ground to a fatty paste, which contains the cocoa butter, and sugar and additives like **lecithin** and vanilla are added. (In commercial cocoa powder drinks the fatty cocoa butter is removed and starch is added.) Cocoa butter is also used as a fatty ingredient in cosmetics and pharmaceuticals.

In spite of their high fat content, cocoa beans are rather nutritious; they supply useful amounts of **protein**, some **B vitamins** and trace elements, particularly **iron** and **magnesium**. Chocolate however, is high in sugar, a stressing food which counteracts the nutritional advantage by depleting the **B vitamins**. In fact, most chocolate contains more sugar than cocoa mass. Consequently, chocolates are loaded with **calories**; a 100 g bar of milk chocolate contains 520 calories.

Chocolate is a rich source of flavonoids such as proanthocyanidins, which make it a potent antioxidant food providing protection from free-radical damage. The saturated fat in chocolate does not elevate **cholesterol** as much as meat or dairy foods since cocoa butter contains plant sterols, such as sitosterol, which inhibit cholesterol absorption. Chocolate contains **arginine**, and the stimulants beta-phenylethylamine (PEA) and **theobromine**. PEA is a mood elevator, which can explain chocolate cravings and why some people will gorge themselves on chocolate when depressed. Theobromine is a milder stimulant than **caffeine** and is known to stimulate the release of endorphins ('feel good' chemicals in the brain). Its downside is that it stimulates the overproduction of fibrous tissue and formation of breast lumps (fibrocytic breast disease).

Chocolate can give only a short-lived boost of energy because its high sugar content can rebound by triggering hypoglycemia (low **blood sugar**), fatigue and depression. To relieve these symptoms, more chocolate is necessary and this is how chocolate becomes addictive. Migraine sufferers or insomniacs should be aware that chocolate contains 20 mg caffeine per 28 g. Chocolate is also rich in **oxalic acid**, which inhibits **calcium** absorption and promotes the formation of kidney stones in prone individuals. Its high sugar content is very damaging to teeth.

Chocolate is one of the most allergenic foods and can trigger or enhance a variety of allergy symptoms in predisposed people, from laryngitis to asthma. In the author's experience, many chocolate lovers, especially children and young adults, who suffered recurring bouts of tonsilitis, were totally cured when they discontinued chocolate. But even for healthy people who use it as a quick energy treat, chocolate is best eaten in moderation. For concerned consumers, health food stores offer a variety of **carob** bars whose taste resembles chocolate (see CAROB).

CHOLESTEROL

Cholesterol is a form of alcohol (sterol) and is a natural part of our body's cells, especially those of the brain and spinal cord, liver and kidneys. It is also abundant in egg yolks, **butter** and other **fats** and, because of this, it has been much maligned in the recent decades for its part in clogging arteries and causing heart attacks, and the medical profession has issued dire warnings about the consumption of these foods.

However, cholesterol is vital to the well-being of the body. For example, it is needed to produce sex and steroid hormones and **bile**, synthesize **vitamin D**, form cell membranes and insulate nerves. It is so crucial that all nucleated cells can synthesize it. The liver itself can produce up to 1 g a day, when only about half of this is provided by an average diet.

Cholesterol comes in two main forms: **LDL** ('bad' cholesterol), which promotes cholesterol deposits and heart attacks, and **HDL** ('good' cholestrol), which protects the body from these harmful effects. Factors that raise cholesterol levels include smoking, stress, the contraceptive pill, coffee, sugar, sweets and nutritional deficiencies. Levels can be lowered by supplements of niacin, **vitamin B6, vitamin C, vitamin E, chromium, magnesium, manganese, lecithin, pectin** and **DHEA**. Beneficial foods for the maintenance of optimum cholesterol levels include **garlic, onions, aubergine, soybeans** and green **tea. Exercise** is also very important.

CHOLINE

Choline is a lipotropic **B vitamin**, i.e. it emulsifies **fats** and helps to transport fat globules to cells. It is needed for nerve transmission, liver function and **lecithin** formation. The brain uses choline to produce acetylcholine, a major neurotransmitter, which conveys brain cell messages and is vital for learning and memory. Choline reduces cholesterol and maintains healthy liver, kidneys and nerves. It also reduces oestrogen, thus decreasing breast lumps and menstrual cramps. Although choline can be produced in the body, it is now considered an essential food nutrient and choline supplements are known to enhance its beneficial effects. For example, they are used in the treatment of Alzheimer's disease and to improve the memory and learning ability of students.

Choline deficiency symptoms include fatty degeneration of the liver, nephritis (kidney disease), gallstones, high cholesterol and hypertension. Its best natural sources are egg yolk, liver, lecithin, **brewer's yeast** and leafy green vegetables. A recommended average daily intake is about 1000 mg. As a supplement, choline is commonly available as choline bitartrate, citrate or chloride, either on its own, or included in nutritional formulas.

CHONDROITIN SULPHATES (CS)

Chondroitin sulphates are a group of thick gelatinous materials called mucopolysaccharides or glycosaminoglycans (GAGs). These are types of water-bonded, long-chain sugars which are formed in the body. They are found throughout the **cartilage**, collagen and connective tissues and help attract **water** into them, preserving their flexibility and protecting their matrix.

The production of chondroitin sulphate in the body decreases with age, and studies have shown that this decline may result in degeneration of joints (osteoarthritis). Its richest source is the extract of sea cucumber, a marine animal related to starfish. CS and sea cucumber extracts are reported to improve various arthritic conditions, as well as tendonitis, bursitis and sport injuries. CS supplements are now available in health food stores and can counter osteoarthritis by helping replenish cartilage, often in combination with other beneficial supplements such as **glucosamine sulphate.**

CHROMIUM

Chromium is an essential micronutrient which is mostly removed from basic foods such as sugar and flour by refining. Consequently, it is a commonly deficient nutrient in the adult population. It is principally involved in the metabolism of **glucose** and the synthesis of fatty acids and **cholesterol**. It is also the central constituent of GTF, the glucose tolerance factor, which enhances the function of insulin and normalizes blood sugar levels. Chromium-rich diets and chromium supplements are therefore a must for diabetics, hypoglycaemics and for anyone with a high cholesterol level suffering from hypertension. Chromium has also been shown to assist in weight loss and to increase energy levels, fighting fatigue.

Chromium is best utilized in the form of chromium picolinate, which is an elemental chromium that is chelated (combined) with picolinic acid for better absorption. The best natural sources of chromium are **brewer's yeast**, raw **wheat** germ, **meat, shellfish** and clams, but supplements of chromium picolinate are recommended as a safeguard against chromium deficiency. The estimated daily requirement of the mineral is 50–200 mcg for adults, and 20–80 mcg for children. Available from health food stores.

CIDER VINEGAR

Cider vinegar is produced by the fermentations of fresh apple juice. It is both a food and a medicine, being used equally by naturopaths and cooks. It contains a combination of **minerals**, organic matter and acetic acid that provides its characteristic taste and smell.

There are many beneficial effects attributed to cider vinegar. First of all, it is a natural astringent and inhibits diarrhoea. It improves digestion in people with low stomach acid and acts as an intestinal antiseptic, inhibiting the decaying processes in the intestines. It also helps to overcome bad breath, increases **blood clotting** and wound healing, alleviates allergies, increases energy and promotes hair growth.

Cider vinegar does not work in the same way for everyone, but for sufferers of any of the above symptoms it is worth a try. When used as a medicine, the normal method is to add two teaspoons of the cider vinegar to a glass of **water**, one to three times a day before meals. A teaspoon of **honey** added to the drink will make it more palatable. It has many culinary uses and it makes a good replacement for malt vinegar in many dishes, especially salad dressings.

CILANTRO SEE CORIANDER

CINNAMON (*CINNAMOMUM ZEYLANICUM*)

A popular spice used in cooking and for flavouring sweets and preserves, it comes from the inner bark of the cinnamon tree, grown mainly in Sri Lanka, Brazil and India. The powdered bark (sold as 'ground cinnamon') is used as a spice and also to make aromatic infusions.

Cinnamon is a sedative. In folk medicine it has been used in various conditions such as insomnia, menstrual cramps, flatulence and nausea. Cinnamon stabilizes blood sugar levels. A teaspoon of cinnamon a day has recently been reported to prevent or delay the onset of non-insulin dependent diabetes which develops in older age, and can also reduce **cholesterol**.

CLAY

Clay has traditionally been used for thousands of years as a natural cure for various conditions. Ancient civilizations in Latin America, Egypt and China knew the remarkable therapeutic properties of clay and used it as a medicine, both internally and externally.

Nowadays, clay is obtained by digging along clean river banks. It is sun dried, purified, ground to powder and sold in bags in health food stores. Good clay, such as green clay from France or the white clay of Wyoming, is sand-free.

Composed mainly of aluminium silicate, clay contains an abundance of **minerals**, trace elements and **electrolytes** such as **calcium, iron, magnesium, manganese, sodium** and **potassium**, which are all easily absorbed and assimilated.

Clay has an exceptional purifying action. When dissolved in **water**, its particles have a negative electrical charge, which attracts and absorbs positively charged impurities. Clay is known to help stabilize acid/alkaline (pH) balance, neutralizing and disposing of toxins via natural elimination, and helps improve vitality and well-being. It protects from unfriendly intestinal bacteria, which can cause a host of ill-effects such as headaches, stomach aches, food poisoning, foul body odour and fatigue. Clay helps maintain a healthy immune system and cell function, even in older people, revitalizing them without side-effects. It can be very helpful to desensitize hyperactive children whose condition may be caused by intolerances to commercial food colourings and additives. Clay can also support the treatment of most conditions, from carbuncles to arthritis.

Generally, as an internal detoxifyer for adults, 1 teaspoon of clay powder dissolved in a glass of water is taken twice daily on an empty stomach.

Its use in specific conditions however, should be prescribed by a qualified practitioner. Externally, clay is now used in soap, toothpaste and shampoo. It is also used for skin applications such as face masks or clay baths. Its application absorbs impurities, promoting deep cleansing and improved circulation, resulting in younger-looking skin. Several clinics and sanatoriums in France and Germany provide a clay cure.

COBALT

Cobalt is an essential trace element in **vitamin B12**, which stimulates the production of red blood cells and is needed in minute amounts measured in micrograms. Cobalt is abundant in animal foods, **meat**, dairy and seafood, and particularly in shrimp, scallops and cod. Cobalt intake can be a problem only in strict **vegetarians** or **vegans**, since all vegetables are low in cobalt.

Even though cobalt stimulates the production of red blood cells, its use as a therapeutic agent is not advised. Overdose of cobalt can cause death in children and symptoms such as loss of **appetite** and nausea in adults. Cobalt added to **beer** to preserve its foam was shown to contribute to heart disease in heavy beer drinkers.

COCOA SEE CHOCOLATE

COCONUT

Native to the islands of the Pacific Ocean, coconut palm trees (*Cocos*) are now grown in many tropical regions for both food and medicine. Coconut contains small amounts of **B vitamins** and larger amounts of **minerals** such as **phosphorus, iron, magnesium** and **zinc**. Most of the fruit, however, consists of saturated fat, which was once wrongly implicated in raising **cholesterol** levels because of a confusion with hydrogenated coconut oil. Coconut has strong antiviral properties due to its high level of lauric acid, a medium-chain fatty acid which abounds only in human milk. This is now being tested for the treatment of AIDS. The fruit is also used as a tonic for weakness conditions.

COD LIVER OIL

Cod liver oil, which is obtained from the livers of codfish, is rich in **vitamins A and D**, and in **omega-3 fatty acids**. As a supplement, in either capsule or liquid form, it supplies the important fatty acids EPA (eicosapentaenoic acid) and DHA (docosahexaenoic acid). EPA is used by the body to produce prostaglandins, hormone-like substances that help reduce stickiness of the blood, making it less prone to develop blood clots and thrombosis. EPA also reduces triglyceride levels and high blood pressure. These combined effects can significantly reduce the risk of heart disease, and the mortality of those who have already suffered a heart attack. DHA, a fatty acid found only in **fish** oil, is a vital component of the brain, and is needed for brain development, especially during the late stages of pregnancy. DHA is very important for children and nursing mothers since it affects learning ability. It provides an important supplement to a **vegetarian diet**. DHA is also produced in the body from linolenic acid, which is found in linseed oil and **evening primrose oil**. (See also FATS)

Pure cod liver oil has been a traditional remedy for both rheumatoid and osteoarthritis arthritis. The first written reference to its use as the best cure for arthritis was made by a Dutch doctor in 1849, and since the turn of the century modern science has been actively studying its benefits.

Cod liver oil was found to lubricate the joints and reduce the dryness and friction in the joint bones that cause the pain and inflammation of arthritis. Unlike normal **fats**, which are first absorbed by the liver, the tiny droplets of cod liver oil go directly into the blood and can readily reach the joint linings. In these linings, cod liver oil is converted to mucin and hyaluronic acid, two by-products that thicken the joint fluid and help prevent bone friction at the joints. Cod liver oil has also gained a reputation for helping to cure other conditions, such as dry eyes, dry ears, dry skin, bursitis, hair loss and arteriosclerosis.

Fish oils are especially beneficial for children. A recent Australian study has shown that six capsules of cod liver oil a day helped overcome attention-deficit hyperactivity disorder in children without the side effects of Ritalin.

COENZYME Q10 (*CoQ10*)

CoQ10 is an essential nutrient that is found in every plant and animal cell. It is mainly supplied by food and, as its name implies, it is a vital catalyst – a spark plug in the conversion of food to energy within cells. In fact, CoQ10 releases 95 per cent of the energy required for life and, in this respect, a deficiency of this nutrient can cause fatigue, hypertension and heart disease. CoQ10 also has many other important roles: it is a strong antioxidant, protects oxidation of **fats** and prevents brown age spots; it strengthens and protects heart function by reducing heartbeat irregularities, hypertension and angina pectoris.

CoQ10 supplementation has been found to be very beneficial in halting gum recession, one of the main causes of tooth loss. It can also help stimulate weight loss, while increasing energy and avoiding fatigue. The richest food sources of this nutrient are found in beef heart and other organ **meats** such as liver and kidney. Smaller amounts are contained in plants such as **spinach, alfalfa, soybeans** and **potato**. Supplemental capsules of CoQ10 are widely available in health food shops.

COFFEE see CAFFEINE, COFFEE

COLLAGEN TYPE II

Research from the early nineties has revealed a new natural, safe supplement that can efficiently benefit various arthritic conditions. Type II collagen is normally extracted from the sternal **cartilage** of chickens and should not be confused with collagen sold in beauty stores which is neither the right kind nor properly purified.

Type II chicken collagen is a **protein** that is the main structural part of cartilage. The painful symptoms of arthritis are due to damage to or wearing out of the cartilage around joints with ensuing inflammation.

Collagen II helps rebuild joint cartilage by supplying it with the necessary proteins needed for growth and maintenance. Healthy, strong cartilage is the key to pain- free movement and elastic joints. Collagen II was found essential to stop cartilage deterioration and to repair joint cartilage, keeping it strong and elastic. Moreover, collagen II also contains naturally occuring glucosamine and **chondroitin sulphates**, both of which are well known to help repair surrounding tissues of the joints. In this sense, collagen II is a complete arthritis formula, with many patients attesting to its pain-relief ability. Available from health food stores, collagen II is best made from organic, hormone-free chickens, free from any additives and **preservatives**. Collagen II is considered a safe, non-toxic nutritional supplement with no known side effects. Its powder is normally taken in 1 heaped teaspoon 3 times a day before meals.

COMFREY (*SYMPHYTUM OFFICIALIS*)

A perennial plant, which grows widely in Europe and North America, comfrey leaves were often added to salads. Its root, the part used medicinally, is rich in **calcium** and mucilaginous substances. The root is soothing and was used to provide intestinal lubrication while inhibiting germs such as E. coli. It is also rich in allantoin, a substance which promotes wound healing when applied topically in poultices. It can also be added to bath **water** to improve the complexion.

Until the 1980s, comfrey tablets and teas were available in health food shops. Due to its astringent qualities, the herb was used to halt diarrhoea and internal bleeding, and particularly to help heal gastric and duodenal ulcers. However, comfrey was then found to contain pyrroliziidine alkaloids, compounds reported to cause liver disease and cancer if taken over a long period of time. As a result, the free sale of comfrey tablets and teas was banned by the US FDA, and comfrey is now mainly available as ointments, extracts and salves for external use.

COPPER

Copper is an abundant trace element that aids the absorption of iron. It is also involved in many enzyme activities and reduces histamine levels, alleviating allergies. Although an essential element, only very small amounts of copper are required by the body and even small excesses can be dangerous, causing disorders such as depression, arthritis, hypertension and heart attack. Among those most vulnerable in this respect are users of drinking water supplied from copper pipes, smokers and women on the contraceptive pill. Zinc supplements can help to reduce excess copper levels, while the best natural sources are soybeans, legumes, whole wheat, prunes, liver, seafood and molasses. The normal daily requirement for adults is 2 mg. To protect from overdose damage, an upper intake limit was set at 10 mg per day.

CORIANDER (*Coriandrum sativum*)

A small annual plant native to Mediterranean countries, its leaves are used for their distinctive flavour in salads and cooking. However, medicinally, the seeds are the most important part of the plant and an infusion of coriander seeds taken after meals can strengthen digestion and relieve flatulence; it is also beneficial for arthritis and rheumatism. Up to 3 infusions a day can be consumed. Widely available from supermarkets and health food stores.

CORN (*Zea mays*)

Also called maize, corn is a cereal grass related to **grains** such as **wheat, rice, oats** and **barley**, and was used for thousands of years as a staple grain by the Indians of Central America. Its food value and wide variety of uses make it not only one of the foremost crops currently grown in the USA, but also one of the most important crops in the world. Cornmeal, which has extensive culinary uses, is widely available and a vitally important ingredient in the coeliac diet.

Fresh corn on the cob has a delicate sweet flavour which is lost soon after harvesting. It provides a good source of **vitamins A, B1, B2**, niacin, and **minerals** such as **iron, copper, phosphorus** and **magnesium**. Cornsilk, the fine tassel on the top of the corn cob, can be made into an infusion which soothes the urinary passages and acts as a diuretic. This can be very beneficial in cases of kidney stones and cystitis, but to be effective several cups of the infusion should be drunk each day.

CRANBERRIES (*VACCINIUM MACROCARPON*)

Fresh cranberries are a good source of **vitamin C**, as well
as **manganese, copper** and **fibre**. Cranberries are also
rich in anthocyanidins, antioxidant pigments which give
fruits their blue, purple and red colours. In recent years, fresh
cranberries and cranberry juice gained wide acclaim
as a treatment for bladder infections such as cystitis. A
study of people suffering from urinary tract infections
found that a dose of 500 ml of cranberry juice had a
beneficial effect in 73 per cent of the cases. Urinary tract
infections can occur when bacteria adhere to the lining, or
mucosa, of the bladder and urethra and infect it. Cranberry
juice contains components that reduce the ability of
bacteria to stick to the mucosa, thus preventing the infections.
Cranberry juice and tablets are available from health food
stores.

CREAM OF TARTAR

Cream of tartar or **potassium** bitartrate (E336) is a natural
leavening agent derived from grape juice, which is used
both at home and commercially. It is a white crystalline
powder, C4 H5 KO6, which is also used for its buffering and
emulsifying action and for its beneficial antioxidant effect.

Cream of tartar is more suitable than **baking soda** for
hypertensive people on low-**sodium** diets because it contains
potassium, not sodium. It is also non-irritating and better
tolerated by people with weak digestion or low gastric
secretions. Baking soda is known to cause various symptoms
in sensitive people, such as heartburn and dyspepsia. Baking
powder may be even worse since, in addition to sodium

bicarbonate, another chemical, acid sodium pyrophosphate, is often added. Another point to consider is that cream of tartar is required in much smaller amounts than baking soda or powder. Cream of tartar is often balanced in equal quantities with baking soda when cooking very acid fruit to take away the sour taste and economize on sugar. For a better raising effect, one part of sodium bicarbonate is sometimes added to two parts of cream of tartar.

CREATINE

A new dietary supplement in health food stores, recently creatine caused great excitement when studies showed its ability to improve athletic performance. Creatine supplementation was first used by the British field and track competitors, who won gold medals in the 1992 Olympics in Barcelona. Shortly afterwards, US champion athletes began to use creatine supplements, and from there its use spread to the rest of the athletic world.

Creatine is not a steroid or a drug. It is a natural chemical that is synthesized in the body from the three **amino acids, arginine, methionine** and **glycine**. It is mainly stored in the skeletal muscles as phosphocreatine, the precursor of ATP, the body's prime energy chemical. Creatine is a part of a system that supplies immediate energy, and creatine supplements can produce a burst of energy. Creatine boosts muscle mass and builds voluminous, massive muscles, which is a great boon to body builders; it also increases energy, endurance and power, and can speed recovery, enabling frequent increase in **exercise**.

The richest dietary sources of creatine are **meat** and **fish**, especially beef, which contains 2 g per 0.4 kg. Typically, about 2 g a day are normally synthesized by the body and an additional 2 g can come from food metabolism. To increase sports performance, creatine supplements are usually taken in 5 g doses, 1–4 times a day, depending on whether the athlete is starting to load the muscles with creatine or is just maintaining its level. Creatine absorption is greatly improved when taken with insulin-releasing **carbohydrates**, such as grape juice. **Vegetarians** usually have a low intake of creatine.

CUCUMBER (*CUCUMIS SATIVUS*)

A common garden vegetable, cucumber was originally native to southern Asia, but is now cultivated as an annual in many parts of the world. The fruit of the plant can be preserved by pickling in vinegar, but it is normally eaten raw as a popular addition to salads. Cucumber has diuretic properties, which can help to eliminate water from the body, and it also contains an enzyme that splits **protein** and cleanses the intestines. Cucumber juice is beneficial to internal inflammations, such as stomach and kidney inflammations and sore throats.

Cucumbers are best eaten with the skin, which is rich in chlorophyll and **silicon**. Externally, a blend of juiced cucumber with equal parts of glycerine and rose water makes a soothing lotion for chapped hands and lips.

CUMIN (*CUMINUM CYMINUM*)

Originating in the East, cumin is one of the oldest known culinary spices and is used as a seasoning in Asian cuisine. The plant has been grown in Mediterranean countries for many centuries; it was popular with the Romans and was one of the most commonly used spices in Europe in the Middle Ages. The seeds, and their essential oils, are also used medicinally as an aid to stimulate gastric juices, increase **appetite** and relieve flatulence. Cumin is also said to increase milk secretion in nursing mothers. The seeds are widely available.

CURCUMIN SEE TURMERIC

CYSTEINE

Cysteine is an important **amino acid**, formed in the body from **methionine** (with **vitamin B6**), and a major supplier of the body's metabolic sulphur. Its primary source is eggs.

Cysteine has remarkable protective and detoxifying properties. It can protect from radiation and detoxify the liver. Cysteine forms the antioxidant enzyme glutathione, a potent free radical scavenger. As such, it can help prevent age-related diseases such as atherosclerosis, heart attack and cancer, and help treat osteoarthritis and rheumatoid arthritis. Due to its ability to break down mucus, cysteine is also beneficial in the treatment of bronchitis and emphysema. It is thought to protect body cells from radiation, especially when taken in conjunction with **selenium** and **vitamin E**. It is also thought to protect the liver and brain from some of the harmful effects of alcohol and smoking. Hair is eight per cent cysteine by weight and supplements can enhance hair growth. Cysteine supplements are available in health food stores and are best taken with **vitamin C**, to inhibit oxidation to cystine.

Caution: Diabetics should not experiment with cysteine, which could counteract with the effects of insulin.

D

DAMIANA (*Turnera diffusa*)

A herb that grows wild in Mexico and is cultivated for its leaves, damiana is famous for its aphrodisiac properties. It is also a diuretic and a tonic, and is recommended for sufferers from exhaustion, and for convalescence after a disease. Damiana is available in capsules as a supplement in health food stores.

DANDELION (*Taraxacum officiale*)

A wild perennial plant, known for its bright yellow flower, it grows profusely throughout the temperate regions of the world. The whole plant is highly nutritious and can be used as a tonic, diuretic and mild laxative. When prepared as an infusion, it can be used to stimulate **bile** formation and is also said to relieve the symptoms of jaundice and gallstones. It is useful for the relief of water retention and to cleanse the body of poisons. The fresh, young leaves, which are best used before the flower forms, can be added to salads or used for juice. Available in tea bags in health food shops.

DATES (*Phoenix dactylifera*)

Native to the Middle East, the date palm tree has been grown for thousands of years. Available in fresh or dried form, dates are high in sugar (mostly glucose or fructose which ranges from 60 per cent in fresh dates to 70 per cent in dried dates. A cup of pitted dates has 490 calories. Dates, however, are rich in fibre. They contain some B vitamins, especially **folic acid**, and **minerals** such as **potassium, zinc** and **selenium**. Dates are very alkaline and can help maintain a proper **acid–alkaline balance** in the blood. They contain a special soluble fibre called beta-D-glucan which adds bulk to stools and softens them. Dates contribute to a feeling of satiety and thus aid weight loss.

DEFICIENCY DISEASES

Nutrient deficiencies cause deficiency diseases – the reasons can be many and varied. For example, a deficiency may result from poor vitamin intake due to an unbalanced diet, poor absorption of nutrients due to low digestive juices or **enzymes**, crash diets, stress, smoking, alcohol, the contraceptive pill or medication. Similarly, deficiency diseases can have many symptoms: a deficiency of niacin can cause high **cholesterol** levels; **vitamin B12** deficiency can be reflected in fatigue and depression; **calcium** deficiency can cause painful leg cramps; **vitamin C** deficiency can cause bleeding and inflamed gums; and **vitamin B6** deficiency can cause kidney stones, allergies and morning sickness in pregnancy.

To avoid or correct nutrient deficiencies, it is best to balance the diet with fresh unprocessed food, and the addition of food supplements such as **vitamins, minerals**, trace elements, **enzymes** and **amino acids**. Determining specific supplementation should always be done in consultation with a qualified nutritionist. However, for general maintenance purposes multivitamin formulas can be taken according to doses prescribed on labels.

Caution: Some nutrients, especially in higher potencies, can cause reactions in sensitive persons. The use of higher potencies requires professional advice.

DESICCATED LIVER

This is dried beef liver which is available as tablets, capsules and powder for use as a food supplement. Desiccated liver is a rich source of the **B-complex vitamins**, as well as **vitamins A** and **D**. It also contains **minerals** such as **iron, calcium, copper** and **phosphorus**, together with **protein** and **cholesterol**. Desiccated liver is good for anaemia, weakness and particularly in the alleviation of stress. The best products are those made from organically grown Argentinian beef liver.

DEVIL'S CLAW (*HARPAGOPHYTUM PROCUMBENS*)

A native of Namibia, this thorny plant has been found to reduce **cholesterol** and uric acid levels and is indicated in folk medicine for a variety of conditions, especially for gout and arthritis. It is available in health food stores in tablet form.

DHEA (*DEHYDROEPIANDROSTERONE*)

An abundant hormone that is synthesized by the body from **cholesterol**. However, cholesterol levels tend to increase with age, while DHEA levels tend to drop, and this decline signals the onset of age-related diseases. DHEA deficiencies have been implicated in diseases such as diabetes, hypertension, coronary heart disease, various cancers and even obesity.

DHEA is now available in health food shops as a

supplement, and it has been found to be beneficial in many conditions including stress relief, the treatment of diabetes, and the lowering of fat and cholesterol levels. In addition, it appears to be of benefit to overweight people and those prone to heart disease, aiding in the reduction of mortality rates from heart attacks. DHEA is now being researched for further benefits such as boosting sexual drive in both men and women.

DIETARY FIBRE SEE FIBRE

DILL (*ANETHUM GRAVEOLENS*)

An aromatic garden herb widely grown for its culinary and medicinal properties. Both the leaves and seeds of the plant can be used – the young leaves to add flavour and nutrients to salads or soups, and the seeds prepared as an infusion. Dill **tea** can relieve flatulence, strengthen digestion and stimulate **appetite**; it can help an upset stomach. Available from supermarkets and grocers.

DLPA SEE PHENYLALANINE

DNA SEE NUCLEIC ACIDS

DOLOMITE

A mineral rock composed of **calcium** and **magnesium** carbonates, it is sold in health food stores as dolomite tablets which contain approximately two-thirds calcium and one-third magnesium. Dolomite tablets are strong alkalines and can supplement both calcium and magnesium. The tablets can help overcome stomach acidity when taken after a meal or during heartburn. For a quick effect, dolomite powder is preferable, or 2 or 3 tablets crushed in the mouth before swallowing.

In the early 1980s, the US FDA cautioned the public to limit its use of dolomite because of a suspected high content of **lead** in dolomite tablets. Recent studies involving 70 brands of **calcium** supplements indicated that dolomite does not contain more lead than several other types of calcium. However, dolomite should be used by adults only, since children under six years of age are less able to tolerate lead than adults. It is best to buy dolomite packaged under a reputable brand name which declares its purity.

DONG QUAI

A Chinese herb, the leaves of which have been used in China for centuries in the treatment of women's complaints, it has now been rediscovered by the West and found to contain phytoestrogenic components which have a balancing effect on oestrogen activity and a tonic effect on the uterus. As such, dong quai is used to treat hot flushes of menopause, pre-menstrual tension and vaginal dryness. In Chinese medicine, dong quai has also been used to treat bladder infections (cystitis), water retention (oedema) and painful menstruation. Indeed, dong quai has been found to contain coumarins, antispasmodic ingredients which relax uterine cramps. The coumarins in dong quai act also as anticoagulants and vasodilators, opening up clogged blood vessels and preventing platelet stickiness. It is also used to promote healthy pregnancy and delivery. Available in health food stores in capsule form, either on its own or in formulas.

DOPAMINE

This is one of the most important **neurotransmitters**, which are the brain chemicals that convey messages between nerve cells. Using dopamine as a neurotransmitter (dopaminergic system), the nerve cells release hormones needed not only for growth and healing, but also for the proper functioning of the immune system in later life. Dopamine deficiency has been found in some PMS sufferers as it suppresses the fluid retention hormone and stimulates elimination of water and **salt**. Inadequate levels of dopamine have been shown to result in Parkinson's disease with symptoms such as uncontrollable tremors of the limbs. An effective treatment in many cases is L–dopa, an amino acid which is converted in the brain to dopamine (and norepinephrinc).

DULSE (*PALMARIA PALMATA*)

A red and blue pigmented seaweed, dulse grows in flat fronds shaped like mittens, 6-12 in (15-30 cm) long. Grown mostly on the coast of Maine, dulse is exceptionally high in **iodine** content, and is also rich in **manganese**. Increasingly available in health food shops in its dried form, dulse is used in soups and stews. It can also be toasted in the oven and used as a chewy snack with a distinctive sea flavour. It is claimed to induce sweating and treat seasickness. A normal daily dosage of dulse is up to 15 g.

E

ECHINACEA (*ECHINACEA ANGUSTIFOLIA*)

A perennial herb native to North America, echinacea was traditionally used by the American Indians for a variety of conditions, from colds to snake bites. It was considered to be a blood purifier, analgesic and antiseptic. Another variety, *Echinacea purpurea*, was used in Europe for similar purposes.

The root, flowers and leaves of the plant contain many ingredients that boost the activity of the immune system, and it is this property that enables echinacea to be helpful in such a variety of conditions. For instance, it can help build up resistance to colds and infections, and has been found to increase the number and activity of the white blood cells of the immune system which fight cancer cells. Due to its wide-ranging effects on the immune system, echinacea is also recommended in cases of herpes, throat infections, vaginal yeast infections, urinary tract infections, inflammatory diseases and bronchitis. The herb has recently become increasingly popular and is now available as a supplement in health food stores.

Caution: Echinacea should not be used by people with auto-immune diseases such as multiple sclerosis, rheumatoid arthritis and HIV. Taken continuously for extended periods may prove counter-productive by suppressing the immune system.

EGGPLANT SEE AUBERGINE

EGGS

Eggs furnish more nutrients per **calorie** than any other animal food except **milk**. Eggs contain about 73 per cent **water**, 6 g **protein**, 5.7 g fat and 0.4 g **carbohydrates**.

Eggs are considered the most nearly perfect source of utilized protein. Eggs are low in fat, rich in **vitamin A**, low in calories and economical. They contain an outstandingly balanced nutrition with many **B vitamins (B1, B2, B6, B12**, niacin and **pantothenic acid**), and many **minerals** and trace elements like **iron, zinc, selenium, phosphorus, calcium, magnesium, potassium** and especially sulphur. Egg yolk is a rich source of the important sulphur-containing **amino acids, cysteine** and methionine, which help build up immunity against disease.

For many years eggs were maligned as contributing to an elevated **cholesterol** level. It is true that egg yolks contain 275 mg of cholesterol but this is balanced by an abundance of **lecithin** (1,700 mg), which emulsifies cholesterol, and a vast number of other nutrients that help metabolize it. The only people who should avoid eggs are those with the condition known as hyperlipoproteinemia who should avoid all cholesterol-containing foods.

Caution: Raw egg white contains avidin, a protein which binds the **B vitamin biotin** and prevents its absorption.

ELDER, BLACK ELDER (*SAMBUCUS NIGRA*)

This small deciduous tree, which is native to Europe, is instantly recognizable in early summer for its masses of pungent white flowers which later develop into small black berries. The leaves, blossoms, root and berries of the elder have all had their uses in European folk medicine for centuries. Elder contains an abundance of active ingredients such as flavonoids, alkaloids and glycosides, which have many beneficial effects, particularly as anti-inflammatories, diuretics, blood vessel dilators, blood purifiers and mild laxatives.

Throughout history, a **tea** made of elder flowers has been used to alleviate lung infections, rheumatism, measles and scarlet fever, and many herbalists still favour a strong elder blossom **tea** to treat colds, flu or fever, with added **peppermint** leaves and **ginger** root. Elder also encourages sweating – a boon in the treatment of colds. Nowadays, elder is also popular as a blood purifier, in cleansing fasts for building immunity and in weight reduction regimes. It is available in health food stores in syrup, tablet or capsule form.

ELECTROLYTES

This is a common name for dietary **minerals** that, in solution, can conduct electricity. These electrically charged particles, which are present throughout the body, are involved in many activities, such as regulating water retention within and out-side the cells. Examples include the bulk **minerals potassium, sodium** and chloride.

ELM, SLIPPERY ELM (*ULMUS FULVA*)

A large deciduous tree native to North America, decoctions of the bark and leaves have long been a folk remedy there for many disorders. Since elm is astringent and abundant in mucilaginous matter, which lubricates and soothes mucus membranes, the decoctions are used mainly to soothe inflammations of the throat, stomach, intestines, urinary tract and lungs. Elm is also highly recommended in the treatment of stomach or duodenal ulcers. 'Slippery Elm Food' is very nutritious and, mixed with **milk**, it is easily digested by people with sensitive stomachs. Externally, elm powder can be applied to cold sores, boils and burns. Elm powder and Slippery Elm Food are available in health food shops.

ENZYMES

Found in all animals and plants, enzymes are complex **proteins** that act as catalysts. That is, they act as agents to speed up biochemical reactions in the body, which would otherwise not take place, or that take place so slowly they appear not to be occurring. Various types of enzymes sustain life in a number of ways. For example, without digestive enzymes, digestion of food would be impossible, and without antioxidant enzymes we could not survive for very long.

Apart from their amino acid structure, various enzymes also contain **minerals** and **vitamins** with which they co- operate as 'co-enzymes'. Enzymes can, for example, enable sugar and fat to burn at normal body temperatures, or combine oxygen and hydrogen to produce **water** in a reaction that would otherwise be explosive.

Each enzyme can perform only one specific chemical reaction, and thousands of enzymes work in harmony to enable all the physiological activities in our bodies, from digestion to wound healing, to take place. The liver itself produces over a thousand different enzymes, but the lack of even one enzyme can break the chain of biochemical reactions, causing imbalances that are reflected as allergies, nutrient deficiencies and **deficiency diseases**.

The secretion of enzymes in the body declines with age, and enzyme supplementation is highly recommended, particularly after the age of 40. Various digestive enzyme supplements of both animal and vegetable origin are available in health food stores. Some, like **betaine HCl**, help people with low stomach acid; others such as papain and **bromelain** are **protein**-splitting enzymes; and **pancreatin** tablets contain various enzymes that split protein, starch and fat for a comprehensive enzymatic action.

ERGOT (*CLAVICEPS PURPUREA*)

Ergot is a fungus that parasitizes the growing kernels of **wheat** and **rye**. Extract of ergot contains several important alkaloids, including ergometrine, which induces uterine contractions during childbirth, ergotamine, which stops bleeding and is effective against migraine if used in the early stages, and bromocriptine, which is used to treat female infertility, inhibit excessive milk production in lactating mothers, and relieve the symptoms of prostatitis and Parkinson's disease.

Caution: Ergot is highly toxic. It contains derivatives of lysergic acid, the active ingredient of LSD, which produces dangerous hallucinations and delusions. It should be used only under strict medical supervision.

ESSENTIAL FATTY ACIDS (EFA) (*VITAMIN F*)
SEE **FATS**

EUCALYPTUS, BLUE GUM (*EUCALYPTUS GLOBULUS*)

A large, evergreen tree native to Australia, its leaves are used to produce extracts and essential oils which are used as a disinfectant in many mouthwashes and toothpastes. Eucalyptus is also an expectorant. In addition, it can be used to soothe ulcers and to relax muscle cramps. An infusion of the fresh leaves rubbed into the scalp can promote hair growth. Can be picked or collected. Available at larger health food stores and herbalists.

EVENING PRIMROSE (*OENOTHERA BIENNIS*)

A tall, elegant annual, its spectacular yellow flowers generally open only at dusk, blooming for one night only before withering the next day. The plant was known to the ancient Greeks and flourished throughout Europe and both North and South America. As well as being cultivated, it can frequently be found growing along roadsides.

The plant contains mucilaginous substances with sedative, diuretic and astringent properties. Infusions of all parts of the plant can be used to soothe coughs, relieve asthma, help lift depression, and also stimulate the liver and the digestive system. They can also be used to produce a soothing ointment for skin rashes. The North American Indians used the plant to treat wounds and infections externally, and coughs and colds internally.

For benefits see Evening Primrose Oil (EPO).

EVENING PRIMROSE OIL (EPO)

The oil extracted from the seeds of the evening primrose has been found to have many beneficial effects, including: inducing weight loss without dieting; lowering **cholesterol** levels and blood pressure; alleviating arthritis; healing or improving eczema and acne (with **zinc**); and relieving premenstrual tension and irritable bowel syndrome.

EPO has also been found to be a rich source of gamma-linolenic acid (GLA). This is a fatty acid which is the starting point in the body for the production of prostaglandins (PGs), hormone-like compounds that regulate various bodily functions. Specific type of PGs perform diverse and sometimes contrasting roles − and their balance is vital for health. For example, PGE1 inhibits **blood clotting** and increases urination, while PGE2 accelerates blood clotting and increases water retention. Deficiencies of PGs can cause many and varied conditions such as heart disease and hypertension, arthritis, menstrual cramps, allergies, asthma and migraines. Available in capsules in health food stores and pharmacies.

EXERCISE

Exercise is a nutrient that money cannot buy and, like diet, has many health benefits. Regular exercise has been found to reduce stress by releasing brain endorphins. It also strengthens the heart muscle and its activity, helps to reduce high blood pressure and high **cholesterol** levels, thus reducing the risk of heart attack, aids weight reduction, relieves constipation, and improves diabetes, insomnia and varicose veins. In addition, it can prevent porous bones and osteoporosis, especially in menopausal women.

Aerobic and non-aerobic exercises have different effects: aerobics involve intensive breathing and tone the heart, while non-aerobic activity, as in a gym workout, increase muscle tone. Exercise, like diet, should be adapted to an individual's condition and needs, preferably by a professional trainer.

F

FASTING

Fasting is one of the oldest-known therapies. Nutritionally, the purpose of fasting is detoxification since purifying the body from toxins and waste substances fortifies the action of the immune system in fighting disease and promotes health and well-being. **Water** is a most important part of the process. At least 2 litres of mineral or spring water should be drunk a day to help flush out the toxins.

The immediate result of fasting is weight loss and well over 1kg can be lost in the first 24 hours. Fasting, however, can do much more than that. It can rejuvenate the body and help to reduce addictions to alcohol and smoking. It also releases **growth hormone** which strengthens immunity to disease. In various Swedish and German health clinics, fasting is used to treat virtually all degenerative diseases, from obesity, arthritis and atherosclerosis, to allergies, eczema and digestive disorders.

Long fasts or fasts intended to combat chemical poisoning should be done under medical supervision. Generally, short fasts (one to three days) do not require medical supervision.

Caution: Fasting can be dangerous for diabetics or for people with heart or kidney problems. Anyone with a health problem should seek medical clearance before fasting. A safer and easier type of fast is the 'raw juice fasting', in which small amount of freshly squeezed fruit or vegetable juice, such as **apple, carrot** and **celery**, are sipped several times a day.

FATS

One of the main food groups, fats are composed of fatty acids, both saturated and unsaturated. Fats are a concentrated source of energy, and are, in fact, the body's energy reserve, supplying 9 **calories** per g. Hard fats are usually from animal origin, and are composed mainly of saturated fatty acids such as **butter** and lard. **Margarine** is a liquid vegetable oil which solidifies by processing it with hydrogen, in a process known as 'hydrogenation'. Liquid vegetable oils, such as sunflower, safflower and **corn**, consist mainly of polyunsaturated omega-6 fatty acids, with the exception of palm and **coconut** oils, which are mostly saturated. **Fish** oils are also polyunsaturated, but contain **omega-3 fatty acids** and other beneficial factors which reduce high **cholesterol** levels and the incidence of heart disease. Olive and **avocado** oil are monounsaturated oils.

They are more stable and less prone to oxidation and rancidity than the polyunsaturated. The type and structure of fatty acids determine the various types of fats – whether they are oil, lard, cholesterol or triglyceride – and different fats have different roles. Fats are vital to the body: they enable the utilization of the fat-soluble **vitamins, A, E, D** and **K**; fats are the only substance that stimulate gall bladder activity, without which gallstones can be formed and they are needed to produce hormones and are essential for sexual activity. Certain types of fats insulate the nerves, ensuring a healthy nerve function. Fats are also essential for skin health and beauty.

Most fatty acids can be produced in the body; the three exceptions – linoleic, linolenic and arachidonic acids (vitamin F) – are known as 'essential fatty acids' (EFAs) and are supplied by food. EFAs are required for the function of every cell, tissue, gland and organ. They maintain a healthy and supple skin and produce prostaglandins – hormone- like compounds that reduce **blood clotting**, lower hypertension and prevent heart attacks and strokes. EFAs also form red blood cells and promote immunity against disease and are essential for mental function – half of the brain is composed of EFAs.

A diet in which fat is used sparingly, mostly in the form of fresh, unrefined vegetable and marine oils, is considered beneficial in preventing heart attacks and cancer.

FENNEL (*FOENICULUM VULGARE*)

A perennial herb, which was originally native to the Mediterranean countries, it is now widely grown in Europe and North America. Infusions of the seeds and roots relieve flatulence, strengthen digestion, help suppress **appetite** and, as a result, aid weight loss. Fennel is also effective in treating colics and ulcers. The seeds and leaves are used to flavour **fish** dishes and the stems are used as a vegetable. Fennel is available from supermarkets and health food stores, either fresh or as a herb **tea** or syrup.

FENUGREEK (*TRIGONELLA FOENUMGRAECUM*)

An annual herb, it is one of the oldest-known herbal remedies. The seeds are used as a spice and can be used to expel mucous from nasal passages. A **tea** made from fenugreek seeds was traditionally known to increase milk secretion in nursing mothers. Fenugreek is also used to lower **blood** sugar levels: in Yemenite folk medicine, it is recognized as a treatment for diabetes – a glass of **water** in which a tablespoon of fenugreek seeds has been soaked overnight is drunk each morning. The seeds are widely available in health food stores and supermarkets.

FEVERFEW (*Chrysanthemum parthenium*)

A cultivated perennial herb native to Europe, its leaves have a strong scent when crushed and it produces clusters of small, white, daisy-like flowers in late summer. Infusions of the dried flowers are a traditional European remedy for delayed menstruation, while studies have confirmed that the crushed leaves produce a good remedy for migraine headaches. However, migraine sufferers should first verify that their problem is not caused by a **food allergy**. The active ingredient in feverfew leaves is parthenolide, which is claimed to relieve inflammation better than **aspirin**. Feverfew leaves have also been reported to alleviate depression and nervous disorders. The herb is available in health food stores in capsule form.

FIBRE, DIETARY

A class of complex **carbohydrates**, dietary fibre is found in many plant foods such as **bran** flakes, whole **grains**, beans, brown **rice, psyllium** seeds, fruits and vegetables. It comes in several forms, including **cellulose, hemicellulose** and lignin – which are insoluble in **water** and **pectin, gums** and mucilages – which are water - soluble, gel-forming fibres. Fibre adds bulk to the diet, thereby increasing stool weight and promoting bulky and speedy bowel movements.

High fibre diets are known to prevent and cure many conditions, such as constipation, hypertension, high

cholesterol, heart disease, duodenal ulcers, diverticulosis, diabetes, colon cancer, haemorrhoids, irritable bowel syndrome and obesity. Dietary fibre can also reduce the feeling of hunger and contribute to weight loss. **Guar gum, psyllium** and oat bran are a few examples of the dietary fibre available in health food shops.

Each type of dietary fibre has its unique characteristics. Cellulose and **hemicellulose**, which abound in foods such as **apples, pears,** whole **grains** and beans, are indigestible and help constipation, haemorrhoids and colitis. Lignin, which is found in foods such as whole **grains, carrots, tomatoes** and **potato**, is an indigestible fibre that is useful for lowering cholesterol, preventing gallstones and colon cancer. Pectin abounds in apples **and** is good for diabetes, lowering cholesterol and reducing the risk of heart disease and gallstones. Gums and mucilages, found in foods such as oatmeal, oatbran and beans, help to remove toxins and regulate **blood sugar** level and also lower cholesterol. (See also BRAN.)

FIGS (*Ficus*)

High in calcium, the fig is considered by herbalists as a healing food. It has a detoxifying action and is one of the most alkalizing fruits. That is, it balances acidic conditions in the body, which adversely affect health (see **ACID–ALKALINE BALANCE**). Figs are rich in mucin, which makes them a gentle laxative for treating constipation. They also soothe the digestive tract, cleanse the intestines and are helpful in the treatment of haemorrhoids. Widely available in health food stores and supermarkets.

FISH

Fish contains **B vitamins** and **minerals** like **iodine, fluorine, cobalt, calcium, magnesium, phosphorus, iron** and copper. Some fish such as cod and haddock are virtually pure **protein**, having no **carbohydrates** and only 0.1 per cent fat. Ocean fish can also serve as protection from diseases such as atherosclerosis, heart disease, high blood pressure and cancer. Indeed, a world-wide study on fish intake and mortality rates showed that fish consumption is inversely associated with death from heart disease and stroke.

Lean fish, under 5 per cent fat, include halibut, cod, haddock, sole, flounder, perch and bass. Fatty fish – 5–20 per cent fat – include **salmon**, mackerel, herring, sardines, albacore and tuna. These fish are also a rich source of **vitamins A** and **D**.

Cold water fish, especially the fatty group, are a rich source of **omega–3 fatty acids**, which can reduce blood stickiness, high blood pressure and **cholesterol** levels. Fish can benefit arthritics, since its omega–3 fatty acids are also strong anti-inflammatory agents.

Fish is a rich source of iodine, known to contribute to weight loss, treating goitre and offering protection from cancer. Being high in **choline**, fish is known as 'brain food'.

The hazards in fish come from water pollution. **Mercury** can accumulate in fish in the form of methyl mercury, which is more toxic than pure mercury. Some fresh water fish may be contaminated with industrial discharge of chemical effluents such as chlorinated hydrocarbons. (See also COD LIVER OIL.)

FISH OILS

Fish oils have long been used by mothers as a food supplement for growing children. In recent years studies have shown that fish oils can also reduce the risk of coronary heart disease and lower high **cholesterol** levels.

The properties of fish oils first became apparent in the investigation of Greenland Eskimos who consumed a very high-fat diet from seal, whale and fish, and yet had a low rate of heart disease. Fish oils were found to contain large amounts of **omega-3 fatty acids**: eicosapentaenoic acid (EPA) and docosahexaenoic acid (DHA). These are long chain and highly unsaturated fatty acids which can prevent sudden heart attacks with a variety of actions: they have an antithrombotic action which prevents thrombosis by inhibiting the formation of thromboxane A2 from **arachidonic acid** in platelets; they decrease blood stickiness, preventing formation of blood clots; they lower blood levels of **cholesterol** and triglycerides, and prevent atherosclerosis; and they prevent irregular heartbeat (arrhythmia), reducing the risk of extremely rapid heart contractions (ventricular fibrillation). (See also OMEGA-3 FATTY ACID.)

FLAXSEED (*LINUM USITATISSIMUM*)

Also known as linseed, this annual herb is one of mankind's oldest cultivated crops. First grown in the Middle East, and then Egypt, its cultivation spread to Western Europe in about 1000 BC and then later to North America. It is now grown worldwide for both **fibre** and oil production.

The seeds of the plant are used for medicinal purposes. A traditional treatment for constipation is to eat one to two tablespoons of ripe whole seeds, which have previously been soaked or ground, with plenty of **water**. The seeds swell up in the intestines and encourage bowel movements. A decoction of the seeds can be soothing to the digestive tract, and can also be used for respiratory and urinary disorders.

Linseed oil is the richest source of **omega-3 fatty acids**, linoleic acid and alpha-linolenic acid. These **essential fatty acids** (EFAs) are vitally important for strengthening immunity and preventing many degenerative conditions such as heart disease. Taking a tablespoonful of linseed oil and then lying down for half an hour is reputed to help with the elimination of gallstones. Available from health food stores and herbalists.

FLUORINE

Fluorine is a non-metallic essential trace element, which is concentrated in trace amounts in the bones and teeth. In its natural form, it occurs as **calcium** fluoride and **sodium** fluoride (used for fluoridating drinking **water**). Fluorine builds strong, hard bones and teeth. Its deficiency can cause tooth decay in children and fractured hips in the elderly. **Tea** is a good dietary source of fluorine.

Although small amounts of fluorine are important, excesses can be harmful. Excess fluorine neutralizes important **enzymes** and interferes with calcium absorption, creating calcium deficiencies, which can cause mottled teeth, brittle bones and nervousness. A fluorinated drinking **water** supply should contain no more than 1 part per million (ppm), since a concentration of over 2 ppm converts fluorine from friend to foe. Brushing teeth with fluorinated toothpaste should be done carefully to avoid

swallowing the paste. Estimated adequate daily intakes are:
adults 1.5–4 mg; children 1.5–2 mg.

Caution: An intake of 20 mg fluorine or over is toxic.

FOLIC ACID

Folic acid, or folacin, is one of the water-soluble **B vitamins**
which are partly synthesized by the intestinal flora. Although its
requirements are low and measured in micrograms, folic acid
is a very important vitamin. Together with **vitamin B12**, it is
crucial to the production of red blood cells, preventing anaemia,
and for the synthesis of **nucleic acids** (DNA), ensuring proper
cell division. It is especially critical to the development of
nerves in the foetus, and a deficiency in pregnant women is
linked to birth defects such as spina bifida.

However, folic acid has many other beneficial effects, in
that it stimulates stomach secretions and improves digestion,
increases oestrogen levels and improves lactation, promotes
mental and emotional health, helps the body to produce
brain **neurotransmitters** (chemicals that transmit messages
between nerve cells), and raises histamine levels, thereby
benefiting nervous disorders.

The typical Western diet is normally deficient in folic
acid as it is easily destroyed in the body by such antagonists as
antibiotics, alcohol, contraceptive pills and anticonvulsant
drugs. Pregnant and lactating women, as well as women on the
pill, are particularly vulnerable to a deficiency of the vitamin
and should take folic acid supplements.

The symptoms of folic acid deficiency include megaloblastic
anaemia, depression, psychosis and epileptic fits, atherosclerosis,
osteoporosis, acne, lack of **appetite** and sore tongue. Folic acid
received its name from the Latin 'folium', meaning foliage,

and, in fact, some of its best natural sources include leafy green vegetables such as **spinach, kale** and **beet** greens. Other sources include **brewer's yeast**, soya flour, **wheat** germ, beans, **asparagus**, liver, egg yolk, whole **grains** and **avocados**. The Recommended Daily Allowance of folic acid is 200 mcg for adults, 100 mcg for children and 400 mcg for pregnant women.

Caution: Excess folic acid supplementation can mask the anaemia caused by **B12** deficiency since both vitamins are closely related. These two vitamins are therefore best taken simultaneously.

FOOD ALLERGIES SEE ALLERGIES, FOOD

FOOD COMBINATION

Correct food combinations are regarded by nutritionists as the simplest and the best way to prevent many common ailments. For instance, they are particularly beneficial to people with sensitive digestion as correct food combinations have been found to prevent stomach acidity, heartburn, bloating, indigestion, constipation and headaches. They can also alleviate allergies, calm nervousness and contribute to weight loss without dieting.

The principle behind food combination is that different groups of foods require different **enzymes** and chemical environments for proper digestion and absorption. If, at the same meal, the body is presented with a range of ingredients each with differing requirements, it becomes confused and is not fully able to supply all the enzymes and secretions at the right time. The result can be fermentation, with all its associated discomforts.

For correct digestion, **protein** foods require an acid medium and proteolytic enzymes, as supplied by the stomach, while starches require an alkaline medium with starch-splitting enzymes, as supplied by the intestines. **Fats** and oils are digested slowly, mostly in the intestines, and do not interfere much with either protein or starch digestion. Sugars are the quickest to digest; some are even absorbed in the stomach, while most are absorbed through the intestines.

All this means that proteins and starches make a poor combination and should not be eaten together at the same meal as they require different chemical environments and digestive processes. On the other hand, proteins and fats, or starches and **fats**, may be eaten together since their digestion does not interfere with one another, but proteins should be eaten only with acid fruits, such as **oranges** and **grapefruits**. Sweet fruits are best eaten with starches and, although sugars can be eaten with starches, they are best eaten on their own as they are absorbed very quickly.

Green vegetables and non-starchy vegetables, such as **avocado, aubergine** and **squashes**, are neutral and can be eaten with both protein and starch meals.

People with sensitive digestions may find that eating simple meals, with as few foods as possible, will alleviate their discomforts and contribute most to their well-being. (See also *Complete Nutrition*.)

FOOD IRRADIATION

Food irradiation is used to preserve foods. Irradiation started in 1963 in the USA, when permission was given to irradiate **wheat** and wheat flour. Its main purpose was to destroy germs and insects that spoil wheat, and inhibit ripening or sprouting. In later years, many foods were irradiated, including **potato**, spices, **teas**, pork, poultry, fruits and vegetables.

During irradiation, foods are exposed to extremely strong radioactive gamma rays provided by **cobalt**-60 or caesium-137. Although irradiation does not make the food itself radioactive, it does cause chemical changes in it, and increasing concern has been expressed on the potential hazards of irradiation. The process disrupts molecule bonds, which can recombine with other molecules, and this can produce new substances called radiolytic products, which poses a question of safety since they are impossible to test. For example, some **amino acids (protein)** and carbohydrate groups break down and enzyme action is modified. There is also increasing evidence that irradiation destroys certain nutrients in the food such as **vitamins A, B, C, E** and **K**.

Food irradiation has been banned or severely restricted in many countries, including Britain, Germany, Denmark, Sweden, Australia and New Zealand.

FOOD PYRAMID

The Food Guide Pyramid is a guide to daily food choices that was compiled by the US Department of Agriculture (USDA) in 1992. It reflects the need for an increased consumption of vegetables, fruit grain and **fibre** and replaces the former dietary guidelines of the Basic Four Food Groups which promoted animal **protein** and fat.

USDA has acknowledged that, due to over-reliance on convenience foods, Western populations tend to be overfed but undernourished, consuming far more fat and far less fresh fruit and vegetables than is desirable. As a result, the West is plagued by the many degenerative diseases of ageing, such as heart disease, cancer and arthritis, which are scarcely found in the Asian countries with their higher consumption of fruit and vegetables.

The food pyramid contains at its base – the widest part – the starchy group, with a recommended 6–11 daily servings of bread, cereal, **rice** and pasta. The next narrowest part of the pyramid is divided into two groups: the fruit group with 2–4 servings, and the vegetable group with 3–5 servings. Next, as the pyramid narrows, it is again divided into even smaller groups: the **meat, fish, eggs**, beans and nut group with 2–3 servings, and then the **milk, yogurt** and cheese group with 2–3 servings. The small apex at the top of the pyramid represents the group comprising **fats**, oils and sweets, which, it is recommended, should be used only sparingly.

Therefore, in order to meet the new USDA guidelines, one would need to eat daily, for example, one **apple**, one **banana**, one **orange**, four ounces of **broccoli**, four ounces of **Brussels sprouts**, four ounces of **cauliflower** and 113 g of **spinach**. Unfortunately, few of us actually eat accordingly, but we should become more conscious of the fact that it is vitally important to increase our resistance to disease by the use of the health-promoting dietary nutrients found in fresh food. Taking **vitamin** and mineral supplements to bridge the gap is a practical solution, but these will not replace the many auxiliary, non-vitamin nutrients contained in fresh foods.

FOOD SUPPLEMENTATION

Food supplements of **vitamins, minerals, amino acids, enzymes** and other nutrients are becoming increasingly popular. Supplementation serves to replace the nutrients lost in food processing, intensive farming and spraying, all of which remove nutrients from food, making it nutritionally inferior. Supplementation also corrects wrong eating habits and poor food choices, such as occasions when the diet is short of fresh fruit and vegetables, resulting in reduced intakes of nutrients. Our affluent society may be overfed, but, for the most part, it is definitely undernourished.

Another reason for food supplementation is that some people require more vitamins than others. Some burn vitamins quicker, while others may have absorption defects that create nutrient deficiencies. Stress, smoking and alcohol also deplete nutrients. However, this is only part of the answer. More people are becoming increasingly aware of their nutritional needs. The symptoms of mild nutrient deficiencies, such as headaches, nervousness, fatigue, constipation, premenstrual tension and high **cholesterol**, are no longer acceptable as part of our lot in life. More and more people want an optimal feeling of well-being, not just absence of disease — which is the medical definition of health.

FREE RADICALS SEE ANTIOXIDANTS

FRENCH PARADOX

This term describes the unexpectedly low incidence of heart disease found in the French population, whose average diet is rich in saturated fat and alcohol. The French eat 30 per cent more fat than Americans and drink nine times more **wine**, but suffer 40 per cent fewer heart attacks. The French paradox is explained by the fact that production of red wine includes the **grape seeds**, which contain important antioxidant flavonoids, such as **quercetin**, tannins and proanthocyanidins (OPC). These ingredients of red wine have been found to provide protection from heart attacks.

FRUCTO-OLIGO SACCHARIDES (FOS)

These are a new class of **carbohydrates**, that are becoming increasingly popular in health food shops. FOS are natural sugars present in small amounts in everyday fruits, vegetables and **grains**, such as bananas, **tomatoes**, artichokes, **onions, garlic, wheat** and **oats**. They are indigestible and are not absorbed in the body as are normal sugars. Instead, they have a great beneficial effect on the intestinal flora. FOS actually feed selectively only the friendly intestinal bacteria, such as bifidobacteria and *Lactobacillus acidophilus*, but not the unfriendly bacteria such as *Clostridium perfringens*, **salmonella** or E. coli. In one study, a daily addition of 8 g FOS to the diet, resulted in a ten-fold increase of the friendly bifidobacteria.

The use of FOS has far-reaching implications. By improving the intestinal flora and keeping it slightly acidic, FOS can relieve constipation, neutralize body odours and improve nutrient absorption from food.

The use of FOS is particularly important when taking **antibiotics**, which kill all intestinal bacteria, both friendly and unfriendly, causing conditions such as diarrhoea, yeast infections and fatigue. FOS can also benefit diabetics, reducing their levels of sugar and **cholesterol**.

FRUCTOSE

Fructose, also called fruit sugar, is a natural sugar present in fruits and **honey**. As part of the **glucose** molecule, it is produced from sucrose sources, such as **corn**. Fructose releases less insulin than sugar and over a longer period of time, and is therefore used by some mild diabetics as a sweetener.

G

GABA (GAMMA-AMINOBUTYRIC ACID)

An amino acid supplement that is gaining popularity for its
anti-anxiety effects, GABA is produced in the body from
glutamic acid and acts as an inhibitory neurotransmitter
That is, it slows down activity in the part of the brain
called the lymbic system, which is our emotional alarm
bell. Thus, GABA is able to help reduce stressful feelings
such as anxiety, fear and panic. As a natural tranquillizer,
GABA can partially replace valium by binding to the same
brain receptors, providing tranquillization. It is also r
eported to help reduce frequent night-time urination
by suppressing the hormone prolactin, which stimulates
urination. Available from health food stores.

GAMMA-ORYZANOL

As an ester of ferrulic acid, gamma oryzanol is an **antioxidant**
within plant cells that is widely distributed in foods such as
rice, wheat, barley, oats, vegetables, olives, **tomatoes** and
citrus fruits. Found mainly in the **bran** part of **grains,** it
promotes their growth. Gamma–oryzanol was isolated from
rice-bran oil and was first used by the Japanese to treat anxiety.
It is now used mainly to treat the hot flushes of menopause,
high **cholesterol** levels and digestive disorders such as ulcers,
gastritis and irritable bowel syndrome.

As a potent antioxidant, gamma–oryzanol can help to
counter the damaging effects of radiation and chemotherapy.

Animal studies have shown that it can also have anti-cancer effects. Many bodybuilders believe that gamma-oryzanol increases the secretion of **growth hormone**, since it acts on the hypothalamus and the pituitary gland, the sources of this hormone (see ARGININE). Gamma-oryzanol is considered to be a safe, natural substance and its normal total daily intake is estimated at 300 mg.

GARLIC (*ALLIUM SATIVUM*)

Garlic, a pungently flavoured bulb of the **onion** family, is a classic example of a combination of food and folk medicine. It contains various potent sulphur compounds such as alliin and allicin which boost immunity to diseases and which have antibacterial, antifungal and antithrombic effects. Allicin extract in cream form was recently found in clinical trials to kill the so-called 'super bug' (MRSA), which is resistant to antibiotics in treating skin disorders such as eczema and acne.

Garlic is extensively used to prevent and treat colds and flu. It has been found to lower blood pressure and reduce blood stickiness, thus preventing coronary thrombosis, heart attacks and strokes, and has also been found to be beneficial in inhibiting the growth of cancerous tumours, and treating diabetes, yeast infections, allergies and stress.

The long-term use of garlic can benefit people who are predisposed to conditions such as heart disease, cancer or diabetes, or have a family history of them.

As a strong anti-fungal, garlic has long been a folk remedy for children with intestinal parasites such as pinworms or tapeworms. It has also been used in the treatment of athlete's foot and yeast overgrowth. The strong odour of the herb can be suppressed by eating fresh

parsley with it. There are also many brands of odourless garlic oil capsules available in health food shops.

GENETICALLY MODIFIED FOODS (*GM*)

In recent years, genetic engineering has been applied in farming with the purpose of improving certain characteristics in plants. Genetic modification consists of splicing a gene with a desired quality from one plant and inserting it into another. In nature, only closely related plants are able to mix genes, but in genetic engineering it is possible to mix genes of entirely unrelated plants or organisms. For example, a variety of tomato was made frost-resistant by the insertion of an 'antifreeze' gene from an arctic **fish**.

However, there has been concern among many people that once new genes enter the DNA chain, they can cause genetic damage with unpredictable results. For instance, in 1989 a batch of genetically engineered L-**tryptophan**, a calming amino acid, caused the death of 30 people in the United States and afflicted thousands of others with a rare blood disorder. This subject eventually became a public controversy when it became known that staple **grains** such as **soybeans** and maize, for example, were being genetically modified to resist herbicides as these grains are widely used in many human foods and also in animal feeds. Scientists became concerned that GM foods could compromise the treatment of disease in animals and humans by increasing resistance to the commonly used antibiotic ampicillin, which could lead to the creation of drug-resistant bugs. It is also feared that GM plants will cross-pollinate with adjacent fields and pose a threat to wildlife. Consumer groups and supermarkets have demanded clear labelling and the segregation of GM foods, in the hope that the GM foods of today do not become the BSE-type problem of tomorrow.

GENISTEIN

A naturally occuring isoflavone which is mostly prevalent in **soybeans**, **alfalfa** and clover, genistein was recently introduced in health food stores as a natural food supplement due to its significant cancer-preventing effects. A recent study done by Catherine Rice-Evans at Guy's Hospital, London, has confirmed that the soy isoflavone genistein (and to a somewhat lesser degree daidzein) is a powerful antioxidant in its ability to quench free radicals.

Genistein is also a phytoestrogen (plant estrogen) with both oestrogenic and anti-oestrogenic activities, a paradox that is the key to its cancer preventive properties.

Compared to hormone replacement therapy (HRT), the oestrogenic activity of genistein is much milder and safer.

It has been known for some time that people who consumed large amounts of soya beans and soy products such as soya drinks, **tofu** or **miso**, have a lower incidence of various cancers. Breast cancer, which according to recent statistics affects one woman in eight, is linked to higher levels of oestrogen. Genistein was found to bind to oestrogen receptors in cells, inhibiting the harmful action of excess oestrogen or cancer-causing pesticides, thus reducing the risk of breast cancer. (See also 'The Soya Revolution' in *Complete Nutrition*.)

GERMANIUM

Germanium is a much-acclaimed trace element. It is a semimetal and semiconductor, and was once used to make transistors. Nutritionally, organic germanium boosts the immune system by stimulating the production of interferon and other immune cells, increasing resistance to various diseases. Organic germanium also lowers the oxygen requirements of body organs and is a powerful antioxidant, reducing peroxidation damage, and helping prevent the debilitating diseases of ageing. As such, it was found to have a beneficial effect on ovarian malignancies, colon cancer and Hodgkin's disease. Organic germanium was also found to have anti-arthritic properties.

Trace amounts of germanium are present in most foods, but richer amounts are found in **ginseng, garlic, aloe vera** and **comfrey**, which may partially explain the health-promoting effects of these foods. Germanium is also available as a supplement in health food stores.

GINKGO BILOBA

A tree existing for millions of years, its leaves were found to contain substances capable of reversing the ageing of the brain. Powerful antioxidant compounds such as flavonoids and terpenes, gingkolides and bilobalides, which make up 47 per cent of the ginkgo extract, are considered to halt lipid peroxidation in the brain and protect brain cells.

Since ginkgo increases the supplies of both blood and oxygen to the brain, it can benefit sufferers of degenerative diseases such as dementia, which can be a result of poor flow of blood and oxygen to the brain. Indeed, various studies have shown that *Ginkgo biloba* extracts not only benefit cases of Alzheimer's disease, but can also improve short-term memory in students and act as an effective memory aid for all ages.

Ginkgo's ability to improve blood supply was recently

found to be beneficial in other conditions, such as male erectile dysfunction and male impotency, senile macular degeneration, hearing loss in the elderly and tinnitus.

Ginkgo biloba extract capsules are widely available in health food stores. A minimum usage period of three months is normally necessary to achieve benefits.

GINGER (*ZINGIBER OFFICINALIS*)

A perennial plant grown in most of the tropical regions of the world, its powdered root has been used for centuries as a culinary spice and in infusions. Ginger is a stimulant that relieves flatulence, discharges mucus, strengthens digestion, stimulates glandular secretions and relieves vomiting. Blended with **cinnamon** powder, ginger makes a pleasant **tea** and ginger root powder taken in doses of 250 mg four times a day can reduce morning sickness of pregnancy. In some African cultures, ginger is considered to be an aphrodisiac.

GINSENG (*PANAX GINSENG*)

Ginseng is the most widely used herb of Chinese medicine, hence its name, *panax*, which means 'cure-all'. It is a small perennial plant, native to Korea but also cultivated in China, Siberia and the USA. Ginseng is grown for its root which is said to abound with healing properties and which is used mainly as a tonic. Its many uses, however, include treatment for a great variety of disorders, from hypertension, fatigue and stress, to weak memory, arthritis and impotence. The root contains glycosides, called ginsenosides, with **vitamins** and **minerals** that fortify the immune system, increasing resistance to various diseases, and promoting physical and mental vigour. Ginseng is available from health food shops as **teas**, capsules and extracts.

GLANDULAR THERAPY

Eating raw animal glands, such as the liver, is a practice that has been followed since ancient times to invigorate the body and fight disease. The therapeutic value of endocrine glands, which secrete hormones and **enzymes**, has recently been gaining increased scientific recognition, and following the development of safe production methods, such as freeze-drying, which preserve the nutrients of the glands, glandular supplements have become available.

The principle underlying glandular therapy is that 'like cures like'. For example, a person with a weak liver or liver disease can benefit by eating animal liver. Indeed, science has confirmed that extracts of various glands such as those of the thyroid, adrenal, thymus, pancreas or pituitary, are quite effective when taken orally because of their active hormone and enzyme content. **Pancreatin**, for example, is a popular digestive aid made from the pancreas gland, which contains a comprehensive range of digestive **enzymes**. The adrenal gland is rich in hormones and its extracts are used to overcome stress and many other ailments, such as asthma, heart disease, flu, depression, headaches, irritable bowel syndrome, diabetes, PMS and arthritis.

Glandular extracts are now available in health food shops in various combinations, on their own, and are included in multivitamin preparations.

GLAZING AGENTS

These are food additives, such as beeswax or shellac, which are used by the food industry to give foods a shiny appearance or a protective coating.

GLA SEE EVENING PRIMROSE OIL

GLUCOMANNAN

A gum, which is derived from a plant tuber, it acts as dietary **fibre** by absorbing **water** and, in the intestines, can expand to 60 times its weight. It is also a fat mobilizer, combining with fat to removes it from the colon. Thus, glucomannan can be used to treat constipation, curb **appetite**, normalize **blood sugar** levels, help with weight loss, reduce **cholesterol** levels and treat diabetes.

Glucomannan is sold in capsules and, for best results, 2–3 capsules should be taken with a large glass of water half an hour before meals.

GLUCONATES

These are mineral complexes bound with gluconic acid. Gluconic acid is naturally produced by the body and used as a source of energy. The gluconate complex enables **minerals** to cross the intestinal wall and be absorbed into the blood stream more efficiently. Mineral gluconates, sold in health food shops, include **iron, zinc, calcium, magnesium, potassium, manganese** and **copper**. (See CHELATION.)

GLUCOSE

Also known as **blood sugar**, it is the form of sugar that is
produced in plant and animal tissues and is used to provide
energy. It is the end product of assimilated foods, and a feeling
of well-being and high energy levels depends upon the
maintenance of normal levels of glucose in the blood, cells and
muscles. The brain is particularly dependent on glucose as its
energy source: a drop in the brain's glucose level immediately
releases hormones, such as adrenaline and glucagone, to restore
it. A chronic condition of low blood glucose levels is known as
hypoglycaemia, while its opposite – chronic high glucose levels –
is diabetes. Glucose is found naturally in fruits, **grains** and plants.

GLUCOSE TOLERANCE FACTOR see CHROMIUM

GLUCOSE TOLERANCE TEST (GTT)

This is the standard laboratory test for detecting
hypoglycaemia or diabetes. To check for diabetes, the patient
is normally given a solution of 100 g glucose to drink first
thing in the morning, on an empty stomach, and blood
samples are then taken after 30 minutes, and again after an
hour, to check the glucose levels. The most reliable GTT for
hypoglycaemia is one that lasts for 5–6 hours, with blood
samples being taken each hour.

GLUCOSAMINE SULPHATE (GS)

Glucosamine sulphate is a compound that occurs naturally in
the joints. It is made up of glucose, an amino acid (**glutamine**)
and **sulphur**. Its main function is to stimulate the growth of

cartilage, by serving as a building block for its production. GS provides proteoglycans (PAS), **protein** and sugar molecules that attract and hold water, and produces a group of gelatinous compounds known as glycosaminoglycans (GAGs), which bind water in the cartilage matrix and help prevent cartilage from breaking down. GS also promotes the incorporation of sulphur into the cartilage, which means that GS is necessary not only for joint function, but also for stimulating its repair. In this sense, GS works best with chondroitin sulphate (CS) to repair cartilage damage, preventing osteoarthritis. While GS holds water in the cartilage, CS acts more like a 'water magnet'.

In many people, the production of GS in the body declines with age, as cartilage loses its flexibility and thus its ability to act as a shock absorber and the result is osteoarthritis, the most common form of arthritis, which affects millions of elderly people. It has been suggested that GS deficiency is the major causative factor in osteoarthritis and, as a result, GS supplements have been tried and found successful in the treatment of the disease.

GS is now widely available in health food stores as a dietary supplement. Taken orally, it is efficiently absorbed and tolerated with no known contra-indications or adverse interactions with drugs. In some cases of nausea or heartburn, it is advised that GS should be taken with meals. The standard dose is 500 mg, 3 times a day, but overweight people may require more, depending on their body weight, the guide lines being 20 mg per kg of body weight a day.

GLUTAMINE AND GLUTAMIC ACID

Glutamic acid is a non-essential amino acid that has been dubbed 'the brain fuel'. It is usually supplied by food and is the most prominent amino acid in **wheat**. Glutamic acid combines with poisonous ammonia in the brain and detoxifies it, producing glutamine, the actual brain booster. As a supplement, glutamine improves brain function, alertness and mood, and can help in the treatment of alcoholism and migraine, and also to overcome a sweet tooth. Glutamic acid, by helping produce **GABA** (a calming neurotransmitter) in the brain, has an indirect calming effect.

Studies during the 90s revealed that glutamine is the primary fuel for the growth of immune cells, especially intestinal lining cells. It is therefore used now in the treatment of the leaky gut syndrome, Crohn's disease, irritable bowel syndrome and ulcerative colitis. Glutamine is a liver detoxifyer and is also indicated for allergies and arthritis.

A daily supplement of 3–5 g of glutamine powder or capsules is a normal protective dose. Higher therapeutic doses should be taken under nutritional or medical supervision.

Being heat-sensitive, glutamine is best kept in the fridge.

GLUTATHIONE, L-GLUTATHIONE

A potent antioxidant, it is a peptide produced in the body from three **amino acids, glycine**, glutamic and **cysteine**. Glutathione helps to prevent many of the degenerative diseases of ageing, such as heart disease, cancer and arthritis, and it is also thought to increase life-span. This is a result of its participation in various enzyme systems, such as glutathione peroxidase and glutathione reductase, that neutralize free radicals and reduce their oxidative damage. Since glutathione is abundant in the lens, it is especially helpful in preventing the progression of eye cataracts. It also provides protection from the effects of pollution, smoking and radiation and is a detoxifier of toxic metals, metabolic by-products and hormonal waste. Glutathione can thus improve detoxification of the liver by neutralizing toxins and, as an antioxidant, it protects the heart by preventing cholesterol oxidation. Its levels in the body can be raised by eating more fresh fruit and vegetables and by supplements of glutamine, cysteine, **vitamin C** and selenium. It is available from health food stores.

GLUTEN

This is the major **wheat protein**, containing sub-divisions such as gliadins and glutenins. Gluten is high in the **amino acids glutamine** and **proline**, but low in **lysine**. It is also found in **rye, oats, barley** and **buckwheat**.

Gluten is the main allergy-causing ingredient in bread and the allergy can be manifested in a variety of symptoms. An intolerance to gluten is the cause of coeliac disease, which is an intestinal malabsorption syndrome, characterized by diarrhoea, weight loss, bleeding tendency and low **calcium** levels. The only treatment for coeliac disease is the maintenance of a strict gluten-free diet; this is usually high in **rice** and maize, and should be devised by a dietician or nutritionist. Food labels must be read carefully to avoid coeliac-causing ingredients. Recent reports also implicate gluten in gastrointestinal disorders in people with sensitive digestion, and it is also suspected to be a causative factor in schizophrenia.

GLYCAEMIC INDEX (GI)

As the prime suppliers of energy, various **carbohydrates** raise the **blood sugar** level at various rates: sugars like **glucose** and sucrose are the quickest to raise blood sugar levels while complex carbohydrates like pasta and starchy foods are the slowest.

GI is an index that ranks various foods from 0 to 100, each according to its ability to break down during digestion and raise the blood sugar level, whether swiftly or slowly. The GI was developed in 1981 by Dr David Jenkins in the University of Toronto, Canada, to determine the most suitable foods for diabetics. Initially controversial, it later appeared that mixed meals affect blood sugar levels differently to single food items, and the key was the rate of digestion. Low ranking GI foods digest slowly, provide a longer source of energy and prevent hunger pangs. They trigger a moderate secretion of insulin, the hormone that not only regulates the blood sugar level, but also acts to deposit stored fat. Therefore, the GI is now increasingly applied not only for diabetics and hypoglycaemics, but also for dieting and weight loss, for improved sports performance and for reducing the risk of heart disease.

GLYCINE

A non-essential amino acid that, as an inhibitory neurotransmitter, inhibits stress response in the spinal cord, it helps (with **taurine**) to relieve spasms and contractions that are due to stress or anxiety. Glycine promotes muscle tone by increasing **creatine**, a source of high-energy phosphate released during muscle contraction, and its inhibitory action contributes to the prevention of epilepsy. Glycine is also reported to reduce uric acid levels, thus benefiting gout, and it is involved in the production of **glutathione**, the important antioxidant enzyme. As a major component of collagen, glycine can enhance the repair of injured tissue and wound healing. Available at health food stores.

GOJI BERRY (*LYCIUM BARMARUM*)

Also known as wolfberry and originating from China, goji berries have been used in traditional Chinese medicine for centuries to treat various conditions such as kidney problems, diabetes, high cholesterol level, low energy and skin conditions. Indeed, the berries contain a wealth of nutrients. They include 18 amino acids, 11 minerals, 6 vitamins, 8 polysaccharides, 5 unsaturated fatty acids, phytosterols and carotenoids. They contain more protein than meat and more iron than spinach. The shrivelled berries have become increasingly popular in the West since 2001, when celebrities such as Madonna began to use them. They were alleged to have a strong antioxidant activity, to boost the immune system and brain function, protect from heart disease and cancer and increase longevity. Yet, the medical evidence to confi m these claims, so far, is still scientifically inconclusive; some evidence of the berries health benefits in China came from studies using extracts of the fruit in high concentrations, rather than the fruit itself.

GOTU-KOLA (*HYDROCOTYLE ASIATICA, CENTELLA ASIATICA*)

A native of India and Asia, gotu-kola is a mildly bitter herb that stimulates the central nervous system. It contains several active ingredients, such as saponins and triterpenes, which are known to improve memory and learning ability and, in addition, the herb is now being used to alleviate fatigue and depression, increase sex drive, treat rheumatism, increase urination, treat heart conditions and accelerate the healing of wounds. In Europe, gotu-kola is used to promote the self-healing of skin ulcerations or bedsores from prolonged confinement to bed. In addition, in combination with cayenne and **ginger**, gotu-kola has been found to be an effective energy booster. This combination can be found in health food shops under different brand names, while gotukola is available on its own in capsules containing the powdered herb. A normal daily dose of the extract is 120 mg.

Caution: Not recommended for pregnant women or anyone with a thyroid problem.

GRAINS

Grains are a primary nutritional source of complex **carbohydrates**, which are mainly starch. Whole grains, and their products, also contain large amounts of **fibre, vitamins** and **minerals**, and as such are valuable as a nutritious source of energy. This food category includes **wheat, barley, buckwheat, corn, rice, millet, oats, rye**, triticale, **amaranth** and **quinoa**.

GRAPEFRUIT (*Citrus x paradisi*)

A citrus fruit, rich in **vitamin A** and **C**, the grapefruit contains smaller amounts of **minerals** such as **calcium, phosphorus** and **potassium**. The grapefruit comes in both white and pink varieties, but the pink variety has over five times the amount of vitamin A than its white counterpart. Juice from the fresh grapefruit harvested in September-October is the richest in vitamin C, and is beneficial in colds and fevers.

Grapefruit peel (rind) is rich in **bioflavonoids**, and has a pungent, bitter-sweet flavour. The bioflavonoid activity of the peel, combined with its vitamin C content, is useful in strengthening weak gums, arteries and capillaries. To extract the properties of the peel, a **tea** can be prepared by simmering fresh or dried peel for 20 minutes. Externally, a compress of this **tea** can be used to treat frostbite by helping to restore circulation. The bitter grapefruit seeds, especially the grapefruit seed extract (GSE), are known as a natural antibiotic and antiseptic and to inhibit bacteria, viruses and mould. As such, it is used as a mould inhibitor in various foods. GSE contains many beneficial elements such as **bioflavonoids**, saccharides and phenolic acids, and is used for colds and flu, sore throats, parasites and yeast infections. It is also used to relieve indigestion and treat gastrointestinal upsets. Available as capsules, tablets and powder for external use.

GRAPES (*VITIS*)

Grapes contain valuable cell salts, which are known to purify the blood, benefit kidneys and liver, and strengthen the immune response. Grapes also contain important polyphenolic antioxidants such as **bioflavonoids** and proanthocyanidins, and are an abundant source of resveratrol, a potent antioxidant compound. Various studies in recent years have shown that resveratrol can protect against heart disease, thrombosis and cancer, prevent liver damage and even improve depression. As a phytoestrogen, resveratrol was shown to inhibit the growth of breast cancer and reduce hot flushes of menopause. Grapes are diuretic (reduce water retention) and the dark varieties are beneficial for anaemia. Traditionally, they were used to treat arthritis. Grape juice can be helpful for liver conditions such as hepatitis and jaundice. The so-called 'grape cure' is a form of **fasting**, normally lasting a week to 10 days, during which only grapes and grape juice are consumed. Proponents of this therapy claim that, by its purifying effects, this regime is very beneficial for a wide variety of conditions as it rejuvenates the body and fortifies the immune system.

GRAPE SEED EXTRACT

Grape seeds are one of the richest sources of plant **flavonoids** known as oligomeric proanthocyanidins, or OPCs, which include **quercetin**, tannins and resveratrol. These OPCs, which are polyphenolic compounds, are the precursors of anthocyanins, which are the reddish-purple colouring in the skin of grapes.

OPCs are potent **antioxidants**. They protect the body from free radicals which damage cells and contribute to thedegenerative diseases of ageing like heart attack, cancer, strokes and arthritis. As such, they were found to be 20 times stronger than **vitamin C** and 50 times stronger than **vitamin E**. Moreover, OPCs even enhance the action of these vitamins in the body.

OPCs are known to inhibit protease **enzymes**, which break down **proteins** during inflammations protecting the blood vessel walls. And indeed, studies of OPCs have revealed their effectiveness in treating circulatory disorders by strengthening the capillaries, reducing hypertension and the risk of heart attack. Research shows that proanthocyanidins prevent the cross-linking of cells, increasing the strength and elasticity of connective tissues in skin and joints, so preventing the main cause of wrinkles and ageing. Proanthocyanidins also inhibit the release of histamine which causes the uncomfortable symptoms associated with allergies and colds. Grape seeds also contain a small amount of catechins, a group of polyphenol fl vonoids which have a strong antioxidant effect and were found especially to protect the liver against hepatitis. Available in health food stores, grape seed extracts come in capsules on their own or incorporated in antioxidant formulaes. Grape seed oil is also available for kitchen use. (See also FRENCH PARADOX.)

GREEN TEA (*CAMELLIA SINENSIS*)

Green tea is produced from the same plant as the common black tea. However, it is not processed as the black tea, nor allowed to ferment after harvesting and before drying, and so it retains most of the active ingredients. Studies, since the 1990s, found that green tea has many beneficial effects It contains large amounts of catechins, a group of antioxidant polyphenol fl vonoids with strong anti-cancer properties, which provide protection against oesophageal cancer and block formation of tumours arising in the skin, lungs, digestive tract, liver and breasts. In addition, green tea was found to reduce cholesterol levels, lower blood pressure, fight colds and p event gum disease and bad breath. New research suggests that one of the catechins in green tea, EGCG (epigallocatechin-3gallate), provides protection against age-related degenerative illnesses, and regular drinking can improve memory and delay the onset of Alzheimer's disease. Green teas bags are now widely available and drinking 3 – 5 cups a day are usually recommended in order to reap its full benefits.

GROWTH HORMONE (GH)

This hormone is secreted by the pituitary gland in the brain and is crucial for the growth and repair of body cells, as well as for stimulating the immune system. It is secreted mainly during the first 90 minutes of night sleep, and also in response to **fasting** and non-aerobic, peak-effort **exercise**. It is abundant in young people up to 30 years of age, and absent, or present in only small amounts, in older and/or obese people. GH has many important functions: it stimulates the growth of immune cells and is well-known to benefit auto-immune diseases such as arthritis; it speeds the healing of wounds; and it stimulates muscle growth and increases the burning of fat to energy, aiding weight loss.

Supplements of several nutrients, taken on an empty stomach, can increase the release of GH in older people. GH releasers include the **amino acids arginine, ornithine** and the prescription drug L-dopa (see ARGININE).

Caution: GH releasers should not be used by young persons who have not completed their growth or reached their full height.

GUARANA (*PAULINIA CUBANA*)

A tall, climbing vine native to the Brazilian Amazon, the seeds or beans of guarana are roasted and ground for use as a beverage in Latin America. Prepared in a similar way to coffee, guarana is high in stimulating alkaloids such as **caffeine**, saponins, tannins and guaranine. It is a very stimulating beverage that is claimed to relieve headaches and migraines quickly. Guarana also inhibits **appetite** and it is used as an **appetite**-suppressant ingredient in various slimming products. It is also used to treat arthritis and to stimulate delayed menstruation, and is reputed to be an effective sexual stimulant. It is available in a variety of forms, including tablets and as drinks.

GUAR GUM (*CYAMOPSIS TETRAGONOLOBUS*)

Originally grown in India as a herb for livestock feed, guar gum is now used both as a food additive and as a health-promoting nutrient. It contains mucilaginous substances which are gel-and bulk-forming, and is used in the food industry as a stabilizer and thickening agent (E412) in the production of products such as soups, salad dressings, ice cream and toothpastes.

Nutritionally, guar gum can contribute to weight loss. It benefits slimmers by acting as a bulking agent in the digestive tract. This delays stomach-emptying and the passage of food through the intestines, promoting a feeling of fullness and reducing food cravings. The gel-forming guar gum also combines with **fats** and promotes their excretion. Thus, it can effectively lower high **cholesterol** levels. Guar gum also reduces insulin levels and is beneficial for diabetics. It is available in health food stores in capsule form.

GUAVA (*PSIDIUM*)

Originating in Central America, the guava is an outstanding source of **vitamin C**, the pink varieties being richer in vitamin C than the white. One average fruit can provide as much as 150 mg vitamin C! Guavas are also a good source of soluble **fibre** and contain moderate amounts of **calcium, phosphorus** and niacin. They help reduce high **cholesterol** levels, can be useful for constipation, boost immunity and protect the heart. They are highest in nutrients when fresh and ripe. Canned in heavy syrup or made into a sugary guava nectar drink, they lose much of their nutritional value.

GUGGUL *(COMMIPHORA MUKUL)*

This is an Eastern Indian plant used for centuries by ayurvedic medicine as a treatment for arthritis. However, modern research conducted in medical research institutions in India found that guggul can also prevent heart attacks. Various studies confirmed that the oily resin of the guggul gum, which contains a mixture of biologically active compounds called guggulsterones, reduces platelet adhesiveness and lowers the levels of blood **lipids** such as **cholesterol** and triglycerides, thus reducing the risk of atherosclerosis, thrombosis and coronary heart disease.

Guggulsterones were also reported to have pronounced antioxidant activity, by protecting the important free radical scavenger enzyme **SOD** (superoxide dismutase), and keeping it in higher levels. SOD protects the heart by scavenging the destructive superoxide radicals and preventing oxidative damage to the heart muscle. And indeed, various studies showed that guggul gum produced a marked reversal of the metabolic changes occuring in people with reduced blood supply to the heart (ischemia).

Crude guggul extracts can cause side effects such as skin rashes, diarrhoea and irregular menstruation. However, guggul capsules, which are increasingly available in health food stores, are made from the purified and standardized gum of the plant and were found to be well tolerated.

They usually each contain no less than 25 mg of the bioactive components, Z and E-guggulsterones. Pregnant women should consult a qualified practitioner before using this product.

GUMS, PLANT

Plant gums are mucilaginous resins produced by various plants, usually as a response to injury. Commercially, they are produced by making a scratch in a plant or tree and collecting the exuding thick fluid. Plant gums are water- soluble and gel-forming and are used by the food industry mainly as emulsifiers and stabilizers. Examples of these are gum arabic (E414) used in confectionery and karaya gum (E416) used in soft cheeses and brown sauces.

HAWTHORN (*Crataegus monogyna*)

A European shrub, its flowers and berries contain many active flavonoid compounds. Infusions, or a few drops of tincture, are widely used in Europe in the treatment of heart disorders (particularly those of nervous origin), insomnia and hypertension. Extracts of hawthorn dilate and relax coronary vessels, reducing blood pressure and improving blood supply to the heart, and are therefore beneficial in the prevention and treatment of angina pectoris. The reddish-blue colouring of hawthorn berries is a pigment rich in anthocyanidins and proanthocyanidins. These flavonoids are potent **antioxidants**; they also stabilize cell membranes and fight infection.

Available at health food stores and incorporated in formulas. (See also GRAPES; BIOFLAVONOIDS.)

HDL (*High density lipoproteins*)

A beneficial, 'friendly' form of **cholesterol** carrier which transports cholesterol to the liver for metabolism and excretion from the body. Thus, HDL prevents the build-up of cholesterol deposits in the arteries, which is the cause of atherosclerosis and heart disease.

HEMICELLULOSE

Hemicellulose is an indigestible **fibre** that absorbs **water** and expands in the digestive tract. It promotes bowel movements and can help to prevent constipation and promote weight loss. It is also useful in the prevention of colon cancer by its action in reducing cancer-causing compounds in the digestive tract. One of its chief sources is oat **bran**, but it is also found in other whole **grains**, fruits and vegetables, such as **apples**, bananas, **pears**, beans, **corn** and **peppers**.

HESPERIDINE SEE BIOFLAVONOIDS

HISTIDINE

A non-essential amino acid that is found abundantly in cereals. Many people are deficient in histidine. It is a precursor of histamine, which stimulates cell growth and reproduction and is very versatile in its actions, from promoting wound healing to stimulating hair growth. As a histamine precursor, histidine has a relaxing effect and can help calm anxiety feelings. It also increases gastric juices and thus prevents indigestion and ulcers. Histidine can also dispel frigidity in women and, in sufficient quantities, intensify orgasm. Available at health food stores as a supplement.

HMB (*Beta-hydroxy-beta-methylbutyrate*)

HMB is an exciting new food supplement which has been found to improve both health and appearance. It is not a steroid or a drug, but a natural chemical that is made in the body as a metabolite of the essential amino acid **leucine**. It is also present in small amounts in both vegetable and animal foods. HMB is a natural component of mother's milk, which underlines its nutritive role. Recent studies have shown that HMB helps to strengthen the immune system, lower high **cholesterol** levels, counteract stress and build strong muscles. In addition, studies with bodybuilders have shown that HMB can increase gains in muscle size and strength by up to 50 per cent. It has also been found to contribute to weight loss. In several studies, HMB has been shown to reduce body fat and promote leaner body mass. One researcher has commented that it seems as though 'HMB helps melt body fat'.

It is estimated that 0.25–1 g of HMB is produced daily by the body, depending on the **protein** intake. Alfalfa and some **fish** are among the richest sources. A daily supplement of 1–2 g is considered normal to obtain reasonable results, and 3 g a day is recommended for athletes on intensive programmes. Since it is a component of breast milk, HMB is considered to be a safe supplement.

HOMOCYSTEINE

High levels of hazardous, pro-oxidant homosycteine were recently correlated to an increased risk of atherosclerosis, heart attack, osteoporosis and other diseases, creating great concern among health conscious people. In fact, homocysteine is an amino acid that is produced in the body as a metabolic by-product of methionine, an essential amino acid found in **protein** foods. In a healthy body, methionine is broken down to the toxic homocysteine, and then, with the help of **vitamin B6** and **folic acid**, it is converted to **cysteine** and the non-toxic antioxidant cystathione, or back to methionine with the help of **B12**. When there is a deficiency of vitamins B6, B12 and folic acid however, the homocysteine is not converted to cysteine but instead attacks blood vessel walls and does free radical damage to arteries. It is also linked to birth defects, such as spina bifida, which arises from defective closure of the neural tube during early pregnancy.

Supplementing the diet with vitamins B6, B12 and folic **acid** can protect against the ravages of **homocysteine**. So does eating more raw green vegetables and reducing the intake of animal protein and saturated fat. Smoking and the contraceptive pill should be eliminated. Methylation, adding a CH3 group, was recently found to be a great protector, by converting homocysteine to methionine. Furthermore, methylation was also found to slow down ageing. And indeed, one such methylating compound, trimethylglycine (TMG), is now available in health food stores in capsules and in homocysteine formulas.

HONEY

Raw untreated honey is a good substitute for sugar and, in fact, is sweeter than sugar and is absorbed more quickly. The colour and flavour of honey vary according to the origin of its flowers and nectar. The sweetness of honey is a combination of simple sugars: **glucose, fructose**, maltose and sucrose. In addition to its sugar content, it contains the

B vitamins and some **minerals** and **enzymes**, and it does not upset the mineral balance as refined sugar does. Honey has been used therapeutically for centuries, traditionally to treat sore throats and coughs, stomach ulcers, canker sores of the mouth and lips, high blood pressure and constipation. It also has a harmonizing and calming effect. Externally, it can be applied to wounds and burns.

HOP (*Humulus lupulus*)

A perennial climbing vine found wild, it is cultivated mainly for its flowers which are used in **beer** making. These secrete lupulin which gives beer its bitterness and aroma. Hops are a mild diuretic and have a strong sedative action. Infusions of the dried herb have a calming effect on the nervous system and are good for stress, restlessness and insomnia. A **tea** prepared from hops will improve the **appetite**, strengthen digestion, cleanse the blood, stimulate **bile** secretion, and is also said to eliminate intestinal worms.

Usually, no more than one cup of the tea or infusion per day is recommended. Hops are available at grocers and are also available in some health food stores in capsule form.

Caution: It is important not to exceed the dosage on the label of the capsules.

HORSE CHESTNUT (*Aesculus hippocastanum*)

A tall deciduous tree native to Europe, North America and Asia. The seeds, which are contained in large, leathery, thorny capsules, known as 'conkers' in the UK and as 'buckeyes' in the USA, have traditionally been used in folk medicine for centuries to treat circulatory disorders such as varicose veins and haemorrhoids. Horse chestnuts were imported from Persia by the Turks who used it to treat bruises in horses, hence the name.

The seeds contain aescin, a complex mixture of triterpenoid saponin glycosides, which has strong anti- inflammatory and anti-oedema properties. Recent studies have confirmed the horse chestnuts's ability to improve circulation and reduce fragility of blood vessel walls. A study reported in 1996 in the *Lancet* showed that horse chestnut extract was almost as effective as compression stockings for patients with venous insufficiency. New studies with aescin taken orally confirmed its ability to assist in the treatment of varicose veins, thrombophlebitis and a heavy feeling in the legs. Externally, aescin can also help in the treatment of bruises.

Horse chestnut capsules are increasingly available in health food stores in potencies of 150–250 mg per capsule. They are made from an alcoholic extract of the seeds, which is dried and standardized to a concentration of 16– 22 per cent aescin. Some formulas also include **butcher's broom, ginger** root and **rutin** for a combined effect.

Caution: Horse chestnut seeds can cause poisoning if eaten in sufficient amounts. It is safer to use the standardized capsules.

HORSERADISH (*ARMORACIA RUSTICANA*)

Valued for the pungent effect of its long, white root, horseradish is put to good use both as a flavouring and as a medicinal agent, especially in Japan. Horseradish contains mustard oil (allylisothiocyanate), which is in fact an irritant. It alleviates colds, snotty noses and sinusitis by promoting nasal discharge and releasing phlegm from lungs.

Horseradish is available as a whole, fresh root, which can be kept fresh in the refrigerator for lengthy periods.

HORSETAIL (*Equisetum arvense*)

A tall herb with a cane-like appearance, it is found wild in Europe and is also cultivated. Horsetail leaves are one of the richest sources of **silicon** and can be used as an ingredient in silica supplements. As such, horsetail can increase **calcium** absorption, strengthen bones, teeth and hair, and promote a healthy and attractive complexion. Horsetail also contains other **minerals** such as **calcium, copper** and **zinc**, and is used as a diuretic and in the treatment of kidney stones.

Horsetail is available in tablets and capsules.

HUPERZINE A

Huperzine A is extracted from *Huperzia serrata*, a type of moss also called Qian Ceng Ta. The whole herb has been traditionally used in China for thousands of years to treat fever and inflammation. Recent studies show, however, that it may help enhance short-term memory and protect the brain from normal ageing damage. Available at health food stores.

HYSSOP (*Hyssopus officinalis*)

Hyssop's leaves are astringent and can be used to relieve flatulence and stimulate menstruation. Infusions of the leaves are also used to improve digestion, suppress coughs and relieve intestinal congestion. Decoctions are said to relieve inflammation. Available from health food stores and herbalists.

Caution: Do not use for periods longer than a few weeks.

I

ICELAND MOSS (*CEBTRARIA ISLANDICA*)

This is a small branched lichen found wild in cool, damp
places in the northern hemisphere. Iceland moss **tea** is
used for bronchitis and coughs, for strengthening digestion
and relieving digestive disorders. It can also help to
stimulate milk flow in nursing mothers. The plant itself is
nourishing and can be eaten as a vegetable after being
boiled for a while to make it palatable. Available from
health food stores and herbalists.

   Caution: Prolonged use can cause liver or intestinal
problems.

INOSITOL

Inositol is a lipotropic B vitamin, thus helping to metabolize
fats and **cholesterol**. It combines with **phosphorus**, fatty
acids and nitrogen to form phospholipids, which carry fat
and form cell membranes. With **choline**, it forms **lecithin**.
Inositol is concentrated in the brain, and supplements
produce a calming effect. In cereals, seeds and **legumes**,
inositol occurs as **phytic acid**, which binds with **calcium,**
iron, zinc and other **minerals**, inhibiting their absorption. To
prevent this, cereals and legumes that contain **phytic acid**
must be cooked, leavened or sprouted.

   Inositol can help to lower cholesterol levels, maintain a
healthy skin and lower high oestrogen levels that can lead

to breast lumps. Inositol, which is best taken at bedtime, can, in daily doses of 2,000 mg, lower high blood pressure and induce sleep. It also has an anti-anxiety effect.

The best natural sources of inositol are organ **meats, brewer's yeast**, wheat germ, cantaloupe, **molasses** and peanut butter. A Recommended Daily Allowance has not yet been established, but a daily consumption of 1,000 mg is advised by many nutritionists.

Available at health food stores.

INVERT SUGAR

Invert sugar is obtained by breaking down sucrose into its components, **glucose** and **fructose**. This is done chemically and enzymatically. Invert sugar is a liquid sweetener, sweeter than white sugar and is sometimes used as a processed food ingredient. It is naturally contained in **honey** and fruits, and it is less taxing on the digestive system than normal sugar (sucrose).

IODINE

An essential trace element, iodine is a constituent of the hormone thyroxine, concentrated in the thyroid gland. As with all trace elements, a tiny amount has an enormous effect on our health. An average human body contains 25 mg iodine.

The influence of iodine, through thyroxine, is felt everywhere in the body. It raises the metabolic rate, helping the body to burn excess fat, preventing the accumulation of **cholesterol** and helping to stabilize body weight. Iodine calms nerves and improves the quality of hair, skin, nails and teeth.

It also regulates the rate at which cells use oxygen, and in this way promotes energy production and improves mental function. It accomplishes all this by stimulating the thyroid gland to produce thyroxine. A properly functioning thyroid is of extreme importance. An underactive thyroid, resulting from iodine deficiency, can cause symptoms such as obesity, rapid pulse, goitre, a cold body, constipation, general weakness, excessive menstruation, low resistance to colds and infections, nervousness and irritability. Iodine deficiency can also increase the risk of breast and uterine cancer.

A study of Japanese women, who normally eat plenty of iodine-rich seafood, has shown that this diet contributed to their lower-than-average incidence of breast cancer.

In cases of underactive thyroid, or when taking iodine supplements, raw vegetables of the **Brassica** family (**broccoli, Brussels sprouts, cabbage, kale, cauliflower,** turnip) should not be eaten. They contain a factor that inhibits the absorption of iodine. People living in areas where the soil has a low iodine content, such as the American Midwest, are prone to iodine deficiency and should take iodine supplements or eat an iodine-rich diet. Some of the best natural sources of iodine are **kelp,** seaweeds, shellfish and **onions.** Available supplements include iodized **salt, kelp** tablets, dried **seaweeds** and desiccated bovine thyroid tablets or capsules. The normal daily requirement is 150 mcg for adults and 120 mcg for children.

IPRIFLAVONE

Ipriflavone is a derivative of **isoflavones** from which it is synthesized. It hardly occurs in nature and was found in trace amounts only in bee **propolis**. Discovered in the late 1960s in Hungary, ipriflavone was initially used as an additive in the feed of laboratory animals. Later human studies however, showed that ipriflavone is plant oestrogen that can mimic the beneficial effects of oestrogen and HRT without their potential risks. Various studies confirmed that ipriflavone can improve **calcium** retention, enhance bone formation, promote the repair of long bone fractures and prevent osteoporosis in a safe way. Ipriflavone was also found to increase the secretion of calcitonin, the primary bone-building hormone. While high doses of oestrogen or HRT are known to prevent osteoporosis, they are also known to increase the risk of cancer. In this sense, ipriflavone can provide a safer complementary treatment. In a study published in *Osteoporosis International Journal*, ipriflavone given with very low doses of oestrogen increased bone density without the side effects associated with HRT.

In combination with **calcium** and **vitamin D**, ipriflavone was shown to reduce postmenopausal bone loss better than these nutrients on their own. Ipriflavone is presently marketed under the trademark Ostivone™.

IRON

Iron is the most abundant trace element in the body. The average adult body contains about 5 g, bound with **protein**. Iron is indispensable for the production of haemoglobin, the red pigment in red blood cells, that transports oxygen to every cell. Without iron, the body cells would 'suffocate' and die. It promotes energy, relieves fatigue, prevents anaemia and increases resistance to disease.

However, iron absorption can be problematic. Only about

8 per cent of ingested iron is actually absorbed and assimilated; for proper absorption, iron needs adequate stomach acid, a deficiency of which is common in the elderly, while protein, **copper, calcium** and **vitamins C, B6, B12** and **E** are also needed for optimal iron absorption. The most easily assimilated forms of iron are the organic ones such as ferrous succinate or gluconate. Inorganic iron, such as ferrous sulphate, actually destroys vitamin E. Natural iron syrups and iron-fed **brewer's yeast**, which are widely available in health food stores, are also well absorbed.

Small losses of iron are normal: men lose about 1 mg a day and women lose much more, due to menstruation and pregnancy. Women, children and the elderly are more vulnerable to iron deficiency: studies have found that about a quarter of British children under five are seriously deficient in iron. Among the best natural sources of iron are liver, raw clams and **oysters**, oatmeal, prunes, egg yolks, brewer's yeast and leafy green vegetables.

Recommended Daily Allowence for iron is estimated at 10 mg for men and 18 mg for women, but requirements increase during pregnancy, lactation, and in any bleeding conditions such as excessive menstruation, ulcers or intestinal bleeding. Excess consumption of coffee and **tea** can cause a depletion of iron.

ISOFLAVONES

These are a class of plant flavonoids found mainly in **soybeans**, but also in other plants such as **alfalfa** and clover. They include **genistein** and daidzein, their sugar-containing molecules genistin and daidzin, and related compounds such as **ipriflavone**, biochanin A, formononetin and ononin.

Most of the isoflavones occur in the plants as glycosides (sugars), but the intestinal bacteria separates the sugar-containing part of the molecule, yielding the more potent antioxidant isoflavones **genistein** and daidzein.

Various studies showed that the isoflavones, particularly genistein and to a somewhat lesser degree daidzein, are powerful **antioxidants** and have significant cancer-preventing effects. All the other isoflavones were found to have a much lesser antioxidant activity and ononin had virtually no antioxidant effect.

Isoflavones are also plant oestrogens. Their molecular structure is similar to that of oestrogen and can substitute oestrogen in the cells' oestrogen receptors. But while oestrogen and HRT have been associated with increased risk of cancer in postmenopausal women, isoflavones help reduce the risk of cancer. In the body, isoflavones are converted into weak oestrogens, about one-thousandth as potent as the body's oestrogen, but nevertheless potent enough to exert beneficial effects such as promoting bone building and helping to prevent osteoporosis.

ISOLEUCINE

Isoleucine is one of the essential **amino acids**. It also one of the three branched chain amino acids, and as such is used by the muscles. Together with **leucine** and **valine,** isoleucine builds up muscle, helps to repair muscle injuries and combats stress. Isoleucine is needed for haemoglobin (blood) formation and for the regulation of **blood sugar** levels. Natural sources of isoleucine include **legumes** such as **soybeans**. As a supplement, isoleucine is sold as a free amino acid, but it is normally combined in a formula with **leucine** and **valine**, the other two branched chain amino acids.

J

JASMINE (*Jasminum officinalis*)

A vine with both deciduous and evergreen varieties, it was originally native to the warm regions of the eastern hemisphere. The plant is now widely cultivated in Europe and North America, mainly for its sweet-smelling white flowers which have medicinal properties. Jasmine **tea** (widely available in supermarkets and health food stores), which is highly scented, has a calming effect on the nerves and can also stimulate perspiration and help to reduce fever.

JUNIPER (*Juniperus communis*)

An evergreen shrub or small tree, it grows throughout the northern hemisphere in countries with a cold climate. Juniper berries are so rich in natural sugars that they are used in the fermentation of gin, which partly retains the flavour of juniper oil. The berries, which are also used in cooking to add flavour, or made into infusions, can stimulate the **appetite**. They contain bitter principles, which stimulate gastric acid secretion and improve digestion, and terpenes (essential oils), which are antiseptic and help to alleviate respiratory diseases and expel phlegm from lungs. Juniper berries are also beneficial for digestive tract infections and cramps.

Caution: Juniper is not recommended for people with kidney problems.

K

KALE (*Brassica oleracea*)

An ancient member of the **Brassica** family, kale is a very nutritious green vegetable. It is a rich source of **vitamins A, B1, B2, C** and niacin, as well as chlorophyll and many **minerals**, such as **calcium, magnesium, iron, sulphur, sodium** and **potassium**. The juice of kale can be used to treat stomach and duodenal ulcers, while the leaves and stalks, when eaten as a vegetable, provide a rich source of roughage.

KAVA-KAVA (*Piper methysticum*)

A perennial shrub, it is native to Polynesia and other Pacific islands where its roots and rhizomes were produced as drinks that were traditionally used as both a folk medicine and for ceremonial purposes. Nowadays, kava is used to alleviate anxiety, tension and restlessness. Since its rhizomes contain kava lactones, active ingredients which promote relaxation without loss of mental sharpness, this makes it very useful for the daytime management of anxiety. In addition to its relaxation properties, kava is reported to increase mental acuity, improve memory, promote restful sleep and reduce pain.

Kava is now available from health food shops in tea bags and capsule form. A normal daily dose is 100 mg and a usage period of four weeks is recommended for its anti- anxiety action to be effective.

Caution: Kava-kava is not recommended for pregnant or lactating women. Its only reported side effect is a mild gastrointestinal disturbance, but prolonged use may cause a temporary skin yellowing. This indicates that its use should be discontinued as overdose can lead to skin rash.

KELP

Kelp includes any of a variety of large brown seaweeds that are found in cold waters throughout the world, growing underwater and on rocky shores; it does not grow in tropical waters. In many countries, kelp is harvested from the ocean to be used as a food, or dried and sold in powder, tablet or capsule form. Kelp contains an abundance of minerals and trace elements, but it is mainly valued for being one of the richest sources of iodine: fresh kelp contains about 100,000 mcg iodine per 0.4 kg, while dried kelp contains nearly 10 times as much.

In addition to iodine, kelp contains **carbohydrates** in the form of both sugar and starches. Its sugar is **mannitol**, which is not very sweet and is a mild laxative. As mannitol does not raise **blood sugar** levels, it is excellent for use by diabetics. Kelp also contains small amounts of **vitamins A, B** and **C** and a substance, **sodium** alginate, that binds with radioactive strontium-90, preventing its absorption and promoting its excretion from the body. Thus, kelp can provide protection from radioactive fallout. Through its high iodine content, it can also reduce the risk of cancer. The high iodine diet of the Japanese, who eat plenty of seaweed, has been linked to the low incidence of breast cancer in Japan.

Caution: People with an overactive thyroid, pregnant or lactating women should consult a doctor before using kelp.

KIWI FRUIT (*ACTINIDIA DELICIOSA*)

Originating in China as Chinese gooseberry, but developed and popularised by New Zealand growers who named it after their national bird, kiwi is a treasure of nutritional bounty. As one of the acidic fruits that combines well with **protein**, kiwi is an outstanding source of **vitamin C**. It provides more vitamin C than **orange** and more **fibre** than an **apple**. One kiwi fruit supplies up to 70 mg vitamin C, which cleanses the body and helps to boost resistance to disease. It is best eaten fresh, right after harvesting, but even when stored for a few months, it still retains most of its vitamin C. Kiwis are also extremely rich in **potassium**, an average kiwi supplies 250 mg, making it suitable for people with high blood pressure or oedema. Kiwis contain **fibre**, mucilage and a special enzyme called actinidin which can help digestion, making kiwis a recommended food for people with weak digestion or a tendency for constipation. Kiwis should be bought firm, but not rock-hard. They should yield slightly to pressure and are best peeled just before eating. Nutritionally, they are best eaten raw.

KOHLRABI (*BRASSICA OLERACEA*)

A green vegetable of the **Brassica** family, it is grown for its large, edible stem which has a slight bitter-sweet flavour similar to turnip. Kohlrabi can improve blood circulation, strengthen digestion and help to stabilize **blood sugar** levels, making it beneficial for diabetics and hypoglycaemics.

It can also help to relieve painful urination, stop internal bleeding, and purify the body from toxins and alcohol. The juice is considered a remedy for nosebleeds.

KOLA, KOLA NUT (*Cola vera*)

The kola is a large tree that grows wild in West Africa and is also cultivated in South America. The kola nut contains **caffeine** and is well known as a nerve stimulant. It fights fatigue and promotes strength, and endurance, and is also used as a heart tonic. Kola nut is used in the production of some popular soft drinks.

KOMBU

Kombu is a seaweed related to **kelp**. It contains a number of **minerals** and is especially high in **iodine**. It is usually available from health food stores as dried leaves that can be added to soups and stews. Because of its high mineral content, kombu greatly enhances the nutritional value of any foods prepared with it. It is especially useful when added to beans and **legumes** as it increases their digestibility. As with any high-iodine food, it improves thyroid function and can help in treating all conditions resulting from iodine deficiency.

KOMBUCHA

A recently rediscovered mushroom beverage, which has been known for centuries in Asian countries and was originally used by Zen sages as a reviving drink,

Kombucha **tea** is now gaining popularity in the West for its great healing benefits.

Although it appears to be a mushroom, kombucha is in fact a colony of yeast and bacteria. It grows and propagates in a solution of weak **tea** and sugar, which, as the kombucha grows, begins to ferment, producing carbon dioxide and alcohol. When the kombucha has doubled in size, it is removed from the solution to start a new batch. The resulting liquid, which is biologically active, is kept refrigerated, to be drunk daily in 185 g doses.

The tea has antibiotic, antibacterial and antiviral properties, and purifies the body by binding to toxins and promoting their excretion. It contains digestive enzymes and valuable lactobacilli which improve metabolism, several of the **B vitamins** and glucoronic acid, a known liver detoxifier. Kombucha cleanses the liver and kidneys, creating several health benefits such as increasing energy and vitality, strengthening digestion, improving skin conditions and promoting a feeling of well-being. Although these benefits may vary in individuals, people have reported amazing improvements in a range of chronic conditions, from psoriasis, constipation and fatigue to thyroid deficiency, hair loss and brittle nails.

Ready-made kombucha **tea** is now available in many health food shops in bottles and as extract drops.

Caution: Kombucha tea is not recommended for diabetics.

KUDZU (*Radix puerariae*)

A Chinese herb, kudzu is a fast-growing vine native to the Orient that was introduced to the USA during the latter part of the nineteenth century. Although it is known in the southern United States as a weed, kudzu has long been used in traditional Chinese medicine for the management of alcohol abuse. A recent study carried out by the Medical School of Harvard University confirmed that kudzu can reduce the craving for alcohol by as much as 90 per cent. Two isoflavone compounds in kudzu, daidzein and daidzin, were identified as being responsible for the anti-alcohol effect. To help in the treatment of alcohol abuse and overindulgence, capsules of kudzu are now freely available in health food stores, either on its own or in combination formulas including factors like cysteine (NAC), lipoic acid, vitamin C and other 'liver friendly' herbs, for a more comprehensive effect.

LACTOBACILLUS

This is the comprehensive name for a group of bacteria in the intestines. They are non-motile, do not produce spores and are acid resistant. They convert **carbohydrates** to lactic acid in the intestines, and are used to sour **milk** and make **yogurts**. The family of Lactobacillus include, for example, *Lactobacillus acidophilus* and *Lactobacillus bulgaricus*. (See also PROBIOTICS.)

LACTOFERRIN

An iron-binding enzyme in **milk** which is also made in the human body by immune cells such as neutrophils and macrophages, lactoferrin inhibits microbial growth by depriving germs of the **iron** needed for their growth. Abundantly found in mother's milk, lactoferrin is part of the protection that breast feeding gives the baby against gastrointestinal infections. Cow's milk contains much lower amounts of lactoferrin than mother's milk and commercial formulas even less.

Lactoferrin slows down the growth of many kinds of microbes and some yeasts, and can also directly kill some bacteria. It also enhances the effect of antibiotic drugs thus enabling lower doses to be used. Lactoferrin is presently beginning to be available by means of recombinant gene technology, i.e., by combining genetic material from different sources. Although so far no negative side effects have been observed, it should be used cautiously until more results are available.

LACTOSE, LACTOSE INTOLERANCE

Lactose is **milk** sugar obtained from the evaporation of cow's milk. As a disaccharide, it is made up of **glucose** and galactose. In the souring of milk (as in the production of **yogurt**), lactose is converted to lactic acid. The milk of mammals contains between 4 and 7 per cent lactose, which cannot be absorbed as such. To absorb lactose, newborns have to secrete the enzyme lactase which breaks down lactose to its components, glucose and galactose, which are absorbable. However, after weaning and growing to adulthood, many people lose their ability to secrete lactase and cannot therefore digest milk or dairy products. This condition is known as 'lactose intolerance' and affects some 70–90 per cent of oriental, black, native American and Mediterranean adults, whereas the rate among northern and western Europeans is as low as 15 per cent.

The symptoms of lactose intolerance include abdominal discomfort, bloating and diarrhoea in response to drinking even small amounts of milk. For people with lactose intolerance who wish to drink milk, the enzyme lactase is obtainable from some health food shops as a supplement.

LAUREL, BAY TREE (*LAURUS NOBILIS*)

An evergreen tree that grows wild in European and Mediterranean countries, the laurel is cultivated for its leathery, lanceolate leaves and fruit. Commonly known as bay leaves, they are used as a flavouring in cooking, but they are astringent and can also be used to stimulate digestion and relieve flatulence.The essential oil (available from larger health food stores in the **aromatherapy** section) made from the fruit and leaves is used for the relief of rheumatism, bruises and skin problems.

LAVENDER (*LAVANDULA OFFICINALIS*)

A native of the Mediterranean regions, lavender is an evergreen shrub that has for many centuries been widely cultivated for its aromatic flowers. An infusion or the essential oil of the scented flowers is a sedative, and can be used to alleviate cramps and muscle pain. It is also used to treat flatulence, headaches and dizziness. Lavender oil is widely used in **aromatherapy** and perfumery. Available from larger health food stores in the aromatherapy section.

LDL (*LOW-DENSITY LIPOPROTEINS*)

These are a dangerous form of **cholesterol** carrier which transport cholesterol in the bloodstream to the tissues, thus promoting cholesterol deposits, clogging of the arteries, atherosclerosis and heart disease. Lowering **LDL** levels in the blood can significantly reduce the risk of heart attack.

LEAD

Lead is a highly toxic element, which even in very small amounts of less than 1 mg a day can be harmful, while larger amounts can be fatal. Its sources in our environment are many and varied: car fumes, industrial emissions, cigarette smoke and lead-based paints in old houses are just a few. Inhaled lead is the most dangerous because it is absorbed in the body much more efficiently than ingested lead.

Lead attacks the brain causing nervousness, depression, apathy, mental retardation in adults and hyperactivity in children. Higher levels of lead poisoning can cause sterility, hypertension and death. Those most at risk are garage workers, painters, plasterers and workers in battery factories. There are various nutrients that can help to prevent the build-up of lead in the body. For example, **calcium** prevents lead accumulation, **vitamin C** neutralizes lead, **vitamin A** activates the **enzymes** that prevent lead absorption and **kelp** contains **sodium** alginate, which combines with lead and excretes it through the bowels. Some cases of lead poisoning have been found to respond to penicillamine, a chelating agent that binds with lead, increasing its elimination in the urine.

LECITHIN

Lecithin is a waxy substance found in all body cells and in various foods. It is composed mainly of two **B vitamins,** phosphatidyl **choline** and phosphatidyl **inositol**, and the amino acid methionine. Lecithin is vitally essential to the body: 30 per cent of the brain's dry weight, and 73 per cent of the liver's fat are composed of lecithin. As a fatty product, lecithin aids transportation of fat throughout the body and, with **cholesterol**, produces **bile**. Lecithin has a remarkable emulsifying ability. It can help to dissolve minor gallstones, reduce the size of the fatty particles in blood, lower cholesterol levels and prevent atherosclerosis.

Lecithin is reputed to be a 'brain food' as its ingredient **choline** is converted in the brain to a neurotransmitter, improving mental function and memory (see CHOLINE). Lecithin supplements can be useful to people engaged in mental work. The best natural sources of lecithin are unrefined, fresh vegetable oils, egg yolks, nuts, seeds and **soybeans**. Supplemental lecithin made from soybeans is available in granule and capsule forms from health food shops.

In the food industry, soybean lecithin is extensively used as an invaluable emulsifier (E322) in such foods as **chocolate**, confectionery, ice cream and desserts. Lecithin lowers the surface tension of water in these foods, allowing oils and **fats** to combine with water. In **margarine**, it prevents water leakage and in breads it is used to increase loaf volume, soften the crust and extend shelf-life.

LEEK (*ALLIUM PORRUM*)

A vegetable related to the **onion**, it probably originated in the eastern Mediterranean region. Nowadays, it is popular in northern European countries, especially as a flavouring vegetable in soups and casseroles. It has mild astringent qualities which makes it helpful in the treatment of diarrhoea and internal bleeding.

LEGUMES

The bean family is a group of highly nutritious foods that is an excellent source of complex **carbohydrates** and dietary **fibre**. In addition, beans provide energy and encourage elimination, and are an inexpensive source of

protein, B vitamins and **minerals** such **as calcium, potassium** and **iron**. From a culinary point of view, they are very adaptable and can be prepared in a variety of ways to satisfy most tastes. Sprouted beans (see SPROUTS), which are more easily digested, provide a rich source of **vitamin C** and **enzymes.**

When combined with **grains** in the right proportions, legumes can provide a complete **protein** that is equal to **meat** in nutritional value. Members of this food group include black, lima, kidney, pinto, adzuki and mung beans, and **peas**, chickpeas, **lentils, peanuts** and **soybeans.**

LEMON (*CITRUS LIMON*)

An excellent source of **vitamin C** and **bioflavonoids**, lemons also contain small amounts of **calcium, phosphorus, potassium** and carotene and, being acidic, can substitute for vinegar in the kitchen. Lemon juice is antiseptic and is a home remedy for many disorders, particularly colds, sore throats, laryngitis, rheumatism, allergies and diarrhoea. It destroys hostile germs, cleanses the blood, promotes weight loss, strengthens weak blood vessels and aids digestion when taken before meals.

Lemon juice is normally used by blending the juice of two average-size lemons with water, to which **honey** can be added to make it less sharp.

A course of lemon juice treatment can dissolve kidney stones and gravel when taken on an empty stomach. In this case, the juice of between 5–10 lemons should be dissolved in water, which is then sipped throughout the day for a period of 2–4 weeks.

Fresh lemon can also be used in salad dressings, as lemonade or as lemon tea, which is made by adding a little lemon juice to a glass of hot water. Lemon rind, too, is very useful: it can be used for flavouring or, if sweetened, it can be eaten on its own as a candy, or with the full lemon. To reap the full benefit of the fruit, it is important to use only fresh lemons, not bottled juice, and to consume them as soon as possible after buying.

LEMON BALM SEE BALM

LEMON GRASS (*CYMBOPOGON CITRATUS*)

A fragrant tropical grass, it is rich in two volatile (essential) oils, citral and citronellal, and some terpenes. It is used mainly for its antiseptic and antibacterial qualities, but it can also be helpful in the treatment of fever. Scientific studies of lemon grass have found the herb to be an effective treatment for flu and cholera. Available from supermarkets and specialist ethnic grocers.

LENTILS (*LENS CULINORIS*)

Lentils are a mildly flavoured legume that come in a great variety of colours and are widely available. India alone produces more than fifty varieties. Generally, however, the green, brown and red varieties are the most commonly used in western countries. All the varieties are a nutritious source of the **B vitamins, iron** and **fibre**. Lentils are the quickest cooking of the **legumes**. They are also used as **sprouts**.

LETTUCE (*LACTUCA SATIVA*)

One of the most popular of the salad vegetables, lettuce is rich in **vitamins A** and **C**, chlorophyll, **iron, potassium** and **silicon**. The darker-leafed varieties contain about six times as much vitamin A and have three times the vitamin C content of the paler varieties such as iceberg. They are also a better source of potassium.

Lettuce can be used to increase the production of mother's milk, improve urination and help in the treatment of haemorrhoids. Lettuce leaves contain a bitter principle (lactucarium) which is an excellent sedative. A large dish of fresh lettuce leaves eaten before bedtime can calm nervousness and induce sleep.

LEUCINE

Leucine is one of the essential **amino acids** fundamental to the utilization of **protein** in the body. It is also one of the three branched chain amino acids and, as such, is used by the body to build and repair muscle tissue. It is also recommended for convalescence after a period of being bed-ridden. Since leucine lowers **blood sugar** levels, it must be taken in moderation as it can adversely affect hypoglycaemia.

LICORICE (*GLYCYRRHIZA GLABRA*)

A perennial herb native to southern Europe and Asia, it is also cultivated elsewhere for its root which contains a glycoside (glycyrrhizin) that acts like a mild cortisone. As it is fifty times sweeter than sugar, it is often used to sweeten medicines and is also as a flavouring agent. Traditionally, Middle Eastern Arabs used it to prepare a strong infusion called *soos*, which was served cool and used to help digestive disorders.

Licorice **tea**, or as an infusion, is diuretic and mildly laxative. It is also an expectorant and is used to relieve phlegm. As such, it is commonly used for colds, coughs and mucous congestions. Licorice is also a soothing, emollient herb that can be helpful in healing peptic ulcers. In addition, licorice root, which contains oestrogen precursors, is used in Asian countries for female problems such as irregular menstruation. Licorice is available in health food shops in powder and capsule form, and also as syrups and candies.

LIGNINS

Lignins are types of **fibre** found mainly in plant foods such as whole **grains**, beans, **peas, carrots, tomatoes** and **potato**. They have various beneficial effects, such as anticancer, antibacterial, antiviral and antifungal activity. They can also help to lower high **cholesterol** levels and prevent the formation of gallstones by binding with the **bile** acids. Plant lignins are converted in the intestines into two compounds, enterolactone and enterodiol, which protect from cancer. They are especially beneficial in preventing cancer of the colon and breast cancer.

LILY OF THE VALLEY (*Convallaria majalis*)

A perennial plant found growing wild in Europe and North America in damp, shady places, lily of the valley is also a popular garden plant. It is antispasmodic and diuretic, but is mainly recommended as a heart tonic that can safely strengthen the heart. In larger doses, it can act as a laxative. Available at health food stores and herbalists.

Caution: Lily of the valley should be used only under medical supervision. It contains glycosides which, if taken in incorrect doses, can cause irregular heartbeat and upset stomach.

LINDEN (*Tilia europaea*)

Also known as lime, this tall, deciduous tree is native to many parts of the northern hemisphere, particularly Europe and North America. An infusion of the leaves and bark is pleasantly aromatic and can be used as a mild sedative. Linden infusions also promote perspiration and are a traditional home remedy for colds, coughs and sore throats. They can also be used as a gargle. Linden flowers produced as a **tea** provide a delicious and relaxing remedy for stress conditions, and it is especially good as a bedtime drink Available at health food stores.

LINSEED OIL SEE FLAX

LIPIDS

A general descriptive term for any group of **fats** or fat-like substances found in the body. This term includes free fatty acids, triglycerides, **cholesterol, bile** acids, phospholipids and lipoids.

Unless protected by antioxidant nutrients and **enzymes,** lipids are easily oxidized in the body creating dangerous superoxides and free radicals that attack cells and DNA, and cause heart disease, cancer and other degenerative diseases of ageing.

LIPOIC ACID

A once obscure nutrient, lipoic acid is now rapidly gaining popularity for its many beneficial effects in the body. Lipoic acid, which has many vitamin-like functions, is synthesized in the body, although not always in sufficient quantity. It is a potent antioxidant and a **sulphur**-containing coenzyme; as such, it is an energizer and plays a vital role in 'burning' **blood sugar** to energy. It is of benefit to diabetics as it helps to normalize blood sugar levels.

Because lipoic acid is both water-soluble and fat-soluble, it is a universal antioxidant and can also enhance the action of other antioxidant vitamins, such as water-soluble **vitamin C** and fat-soluble **vitamin E**. By quenching free radicals, lipoic acid protects cells and helps to prevent the various degenerative diseases of ageing such as heart disease, cancer, diabetes, arthritis, cataracts and Alzheimer's disease, along with many others. It is also a chelating agent – that is, it binds to toxic metals such as **lead, cadmium** and **mercury** and removes them from the body.

Lipoic acid supplementation can increase energy and slow down the ageing process; supplementation is particularly important in later years, when the synthesis of lipoic acid in the body is reduced. Supplementation can also benefit diabetics. Foods richest in lipoic acid include liver, yeast, **spinach, broccoli** and **tomatoes**. However, these foods contain alpha-lipoic acid which is bound to **protein** (lipoyllysine) and is not as biologically active as the free alpha-lipoic acid found in supplements which are available in capsule form from health food stores. The normal daily allowance for adults is 20–50 mg.

L-METHIONINE SEE METHIONINE

LYCOPENE

The red carotenoid in **tomatoes** with an exceptional antioxidant action, lycopene has been found by numerous studies to be a powerful quencher of free radicals, stronger even than **beta carotene** or other carotenes, with outstanding anti-cancer properties. A study published in *Anti-Cancer Drugs* reported that lycopene increased the number of T4 cells and normalized the T4 and T8 ratio, creating an improved immune function. Lycopene is now available in capsule form as a nutritional supplement from health food shops.

A study done at the Aviano Cancer Centre in Italy found that people who eat raw **tomatoes** at least seven times a week cut their risk of stomach, bladder and colon cancers by half. A Japanese study showed that lycopene suppressed the development of breast tumors in mice. Lycopene worked partly by blocking the activity of transforming growth factor alpha, which is known to promote cancer. A recent Harvard University study of various **carotenoids** showed that increased consumption of lycopene significantly reduced the risk of prostate cancer in men. Lycopene, which incidentally is richer in tomato sauce than in fresh **tomatoes**, is also used as a colouring (E160d) in the food industry.

LYSINE

An essential amino acid that is needed to form **protein** in the body, lysine is known to boost the immune system by effectively helping suppress the herpes simplex virus, which manifests in symptoms like mouth blisters and cold sores. Consequently, lysine supplements are now widely recommended for the treatment of herpes. Daily lysine supplements of 500 mg were also found to increase the blood levels of ferritin (an iron-binding protein) in women with iron-deficiency anemia. Lysine is also needed to form collagen, the subskin and connective tissues, and is essential for **calcium** absorption.

Since it is lacking in **grains**, nuts and seeds, lysine supplements can help to prevent calcium deficiencies, particularly among strict **vegetarians** and the elderly. Lysine also combines with methionine, to form **carnitine**, an important amino acid that aids weight reduction and helps to prevent heart disease. Lysine supplements are widely available in health food stores, either on their own or incorporated in specific formulas.

M

MACADAMIA NUTS (*MACADAMIA INTEGRIFOLIA*)

An evergreen tree native to tropical Australia, it was taken to Hawaii in the nineteenth century and the nuts are now an important crop there. They are considered by many to be the finest-tasting nuts and, since they provide a very concentrated food, rich in natural oils, particularly monounsaturates, they are often used as a substitute for **meat**. Widely available in supermarkets.

MAGNESIUM

Magnesium is an important mineral which, together with **calcium** and **phosphorus**, is found mainly in the bones. Smaller amounts in the blood activate hundreds of **enzymes** and participate in various biochemical activities. Magnesium maintains strong bones and tooth enamel, calms the nervous system, regulates heartbeat, strengthens digestion, maintains a healthy prostate in men, prevents swelling, keeps calcium soluble, prevents kidney stones and regulates the thyroid. It also improves urine retention and so helps to control incontinence in the elderly and prevent bed-wetting in children. Magnesium can be depleted in the body by alcohol, sweet foods, and the excessive consumption of milk enriched with **vitamin D**.

Magnesium deficiencies are manifested in irregular heartbeat and heart attacks, jumpy nerves and weak muscles, convulsions and seizures, prostate enlargement, fatigue, bed-wetting and kidney stones. Its best natural sources include green vegetables, figs, **lemons**, yellow **corn, apples** and raw **wheat** germ. **Dolomite** is a natural supplement.

The normal daily requirement is 350 mg for adults and 250 mg for children; pregnant and lactating women need 450 mg per day. As a supplement, magnesium is available in tablet and capsule form.

MA HUANG (*EPHEDRA SINICA*)

Ma huang is the Chinese name for ephedra, a low–growing evergreen shrub native to the arid and desert regions of the Americas and Asia. It contains ephedrin, an alkaloid that has been shown to reduce excess weight in overweight animals by speeding up the burning of fat into energy and by satisfying hunger. Its action is improved when used with **caffeine** and **theophylline**.

Caution: Ma huang has been incorporated as an ingredient in a number of weight loss formulas over the past few years. However, its action is similar to that of adrenalin in that it stimulates the central nervous system, thereby increasing heartbeat and blood pressure. Therefore, ma huang should not be used by hypertensive people or by those with a heart condition.

MAITAKE (*GRIFOLA FRONDOSA*)

A newly rediscovered ancient mushroom, native to north-east Japan, maitake was traditionally highly prized in Japan as both a culinary ingredient and a herbal medicine. Oriental folk medicines used it as an important aid to well-being, to maintain health, preserve youth and increase longevity.

The maitake grows in clusters at the base of trees, and in bygone times it was exchanged for its weight in silver. Maitake contains many important **vitamins** and **minerals** like **B1, B2, B3, C** and **D, calcium, magnesium, potassium** and **protein**. New research also shows that, besides those nutrients, maitake contains a special class of polysaccharides such as beta glucan and, more specifically, its D-fraction. These are complex sugar polymers in maitake extracts, which were found to boost the immune system. Most studies by Japanese scientists, done with the D-fraction of maitake extract, showed maitake to have anti-tumour and anti-cancer properties. Further research is presently being conducted at the Cancer Treatment Center of America to evaluate its anti-cancer properties.

A recent study in New York with a group of hypertensive human volunteers showed that two 500 mg capsules of maitake a day taken orally for six weeks lowered blood pressure. Dr Abram Ber, a homoeopathic physician from Phoenix, Arizona, is reported to treat hypertension with higher doses: 3 g maitake per day for the first week, 4 g per day for the second week, then 5 g per day as blood pressure indicated, since blood pressure is dose-related.

Other studies have demonstrated maitake's ability to inhibit uterine fibroids, counteract diabetes and even to help weight loss without a change in the diet!

Maitake capsules and tablets, as well as the D-fractions, are now increasingly being sold in health food stores as herbal extracts. A significant body of research shows that maitake is the most effective of the other medicinal **mushrooms** such as shiitake and **reishi**. Maitake doses should best be determined by a qualified practitioner.

MANGANESE

Manganese is a trace element with a wide range of effects.
It forms part of many **enzymes**, such as those involved
in sugar metabolism, and is needed to form thyroxine, the
thyroid hormone. It also helps in the synthesis of **cholesterol**
and **fats**, and is important for the production of breast milk
and sex hormones, promoting fertility and male potency.
Manganese was found important in reversing osteoporosis, by
stimulating the production of mucopolysaccharides, protein-
like molecules that help the calcification of bones. Manganese
can be used in the prevention of diabetes and nerve-muscle
disorders and its best natural sources include whole **grains**,
nuts, leafy green vegetables and **tea**. The estimated daily
requirement is 2.5–5 mg, although lactating women may need
up to 9 mg a day. In tea-drinking countries, an average one-
third of the daily manganese requirement is obtained from this
beverage. Supplements available from health food stores and as
multi-vitamin formulas.

MANGO (*MANGIFERA INDICA*)

A delicious and highly nutritious fruit originating in India
from which it has spread to many parts of the world, the
mango is one of the most popular tropical fruits. Mangoes
are very rich in the antioxidant **vitamins C, A, E** and
bioflavonoids. One mango provides more than the
Recommended Daily Allowance of vitamin C, two-thirds
of vitamin A and a third of vitamin E. Mangoes are also
an excellent source of **potassium, iron** and niacin. Easily
digestible, mangoes are especially suitable for people with
sensitive digestion.

MARGARINE

Margarine is made from vegetable oil which undergoes hydrogenation. During this process, hydrogen is added to the oil, saturating its fatty acids and rendering it solid or semi-solid. Saturated fatty acids are not biologically as active as unsaturated ones and they adversely affect cell membranes, leading to various disorders, including high **cholesterol** levels and diabetes.

The hydrogenation process also changes the structure of the fatty acids from the natural type of cis-fatty acids to the unnatural type of trans-fatty acids that interfere with the utilization of essential fatty acids and, in fact, they are not 'recognized' by the body chemistry. For example, they prevent fatty acid transformation to immune cells, inhibiting the synthesis of GLA and prostaglandins (see EVENING PRIMROSE OIL). In the USA and the UK, most of the consumption of trans-fatty acid consists of margarine and shortening.

In a recent analysis of the connection between eating habits and disease from the ongoing Framingham study in the USA, researchers found that margarine, but not **butter**, was linked to a higher risk of coronary heart disease. The researchers concluded that this supports the hypothesis that 'margarine intake increases the risk of coronary heart disease'.

MARJORAM (*ORIGANUM MAJORANA*)

A scented, perennial herb, sometimes a subshrub, it was originally native to northern African and south-western Asia. Nowadays, it is widely cultivated as a popular culinary herb and is available from supermarkets and grocers. Sweet marjoram **tea** is pleasantly carminative. It can relieve flatulence and colic in children – upset stomachs and gastritis can be soothed, both internally and externally, by massaging the abdomen with a clockwise rotation. The essential oil of sweet marjoram is also used externally for arthritis, gout, rheumatism and varicose veins. It is claimed to have a calming effect and can be used to alleviate grief.

Caution: Marjoram should not be used during pregnancy.

MARSHMALLOW (*ALTHEA OFFICINALIS*)

A wild, perennial plant with soft, hairy leaves, it is found mainly in marshy areas and damp, watery places. Marshmallow leaves and roots have long been known for their demulcent, soothing and softening properties, and infusions prepared from the plant are excellent for the treatment of coughs and cystitis, and for soothing the digestive tract in cases of ulcers. Externally, a poultice prepared from the leaves steeped in boiling water can be applied to boils and abscesses.

MATÉ (*ILEX PARAGUAYENSIS*)

Also called Paraguay **tea**, maté tea is a stimulating beverage made from the dried leaves of a South American oak which is very popular in Latin America. The dried leaves are also exported and are available in many health food stores. Maté tea has a high **caffeine** content and is renowned as a tonic and stimulant, increasing alertness and mental acuity. It contains **iron** and is useful in the treatment of iron-deficiency anaemia. It is also a diuretic, stimulating the kidneys, and alleviating arthritis and gout. Maté tea is very satisfying and can help slimmers lose weight. Once made, the tea should be drunk fresh as it becomes black and bitter if allowed to stand.

Caution: People with cardiovascular or nervous conditions, or those allergic to caffeine, should avoid maté. Excessive consumption can cause diarrhoea.

MEADOW SAFFRON (*COLCHICUM AUTUMNALE*)

A perennial herb that grows wild in damp places, but is also cultivated in the USA for its bulb and seeds. It contains colchicine, a poisonous alkaloid, which inhibits cell multiplication. It is used medicinally in very tiny amounts in the treatment of gout and arthritis.

Caution: The whole herb is poisonous and must not be used as a home remedy.

MEAT

Meat is the principal provider of high-quality **protein** and fat with other important **vitamins** such as B12 and **minerals** such as **zinc**. Organ meats, like liver, heart and kidney, are the most nutritious. Generally, meat is considered a tonic: blood-building and helping relieve general weakness. However, its metabolic by-products in the body are very toxic. People on meat-centred diets are often thirsty; they need fluids to flush these toxins out.

More and more studies published in the media are advising the public to cut down on red meat.

With higher standards of living in the west meat consumption soared. The accelerating incidence of heart disease and cancer has been linked with beef consumption, which has increased from 120 kg per person in 1950 to almost 300 kg today. Beef in the 1950s provided more nutrients and was much leaner, with 5–10 per cent carcass fat, largely unsaturated. Today's cattle, intensively raised on high-energy feeds, deprived of grazing and treated with antibiotic drugs, hormones and tranquillisers, have 30 per cent fat. Most of these drugs, hormones and pesticide sprays accumulate in this fat. Meat is often treated with nitrites to preserve it. These can combine in the stomach to form nitrosamines, potent carcinogens that were found to produce cancer in rats after only one dose. Cooked meat has other hidden hazards. When meat is grilled or barbecued at high temperatures, carcinogenic substances called HCAs (heterocyclic amines) are created. These substances generate free radicals, which hasten ageing and increase the risk of cancer and heart disease. Most HCAs are found in fried bacon. Stewing, boiling and poaching meat is much safer: they generate virtually no HCAs. Pre-marinating meat in garlic-based sauce was found to cut down the rate of HCAs. Processed ground meat products like sausages and hot dogs are the most dangerous, since poor grade meats and **preservatives**, which can be used in their preparation, are hard to detect in these highly seasoned products.

Livers of beef, calf, veal, lamb and pork have been known to strengthen the body in stressful conditions. Chicken liver is known to strengthen both liver and kidneys, helping in treating conditions such as iron- deficiency anaemia, impotence, tendency to miscarry, blurred vision and urinary incontinence. **Desiccated liver** tablets are available at health food stores.

MEDIUM CHAIN TRIGLYCERIDES (MCTS)

MCTs are a special type of saturated fat derived from **coconut** oil and are used by the body differently to most other **fats**. In the main, fats such as **butter, margarine**, animal fats and even edible oils are composed of long chain triglycerides (LCTs), which are absorbed into the lymph system and stored for future use. They take a long time to be converted into energy. MCTs, on the other hand, have much shorter molecules so that they can pass easily through the liver and are directly absorbed into the bloodstream. In this way, they are converted much more rapidly into utilized energy rather than being deposited as fat.

MCTs have been found to promote weight loss, increase energy and are also useful for treating epilepsy. They are now increasingly available in supplements and also as MCT oils, which can be used in the kitchen in the same way as any of the other edible oils.

MELATONIN

Melatonin is a natural sleep-inducing hormone secreted in the pineal gland, a pea-sized gland in the mid-brain. It is actually produced by pineal **enzymes** that are respectively activated and depressed by darkness and light. As a result, the pineal secretes melatonin at night, thus promoting sleep. As a natural sleeping aid, melatonin supplements are now commonly used to combat jet lag and insomnia, and to alleviate depression. Melatonin was also found to be a powerful antioxidant. As such, it boosts the immune system by stimulating the production of immune cells, protecting the DNA and preventing the degenerative diseases of ageing such as heart disease and cancer. Lights at night, however, inhibit melatonin secretion. New studies have shown that reduced levels of melatonin, which occur in children who sleep with the light on, or women who work night shifts, increase the risk of child leukaemia and breast cancer. While freely sold in the USA in potencies of 1–5 mg, melatonin is available in the UK as a prescription drug.

MELISSA SEE BALM

MERCURY

Mercury is a toxic element and a common pollutant. Its main sources are **fish**, pesticides, fungistats (which prevent mould in seeds), emissions from coal burning and cigarette smoke. The mercury that pollutes lakes and oceans is methyl mercury, a compound that is fifty times more toxic than pure mercury. Methyl mercury is dumped into rivers and lakes by various industrial plants, such as paper mills which use mercury to protect paper from mould. As a result of this dumping, fish can become a highly concentrated source of mercury. For example, in Lake Erie (between Canada and the USA) irreversible pollution with mercury means that fishing has been strictly prohibited.

A build-up of mercury in the body can cause damage to the brain, kidneys and nervous system resulting in, for example, paralysis and blindness. The commonest uses of mercury in everyday life are batteries, mercury vapour lamps, dental fillings and mercury thermometers. Some nutrients, such as **selenium**, counteract mercury in the body. Among the other protective nutrients are **calcium, vitamins A, C, E** and **B complex, lecithin** and stomach acid, which is sold as **betaine HCl** capsules.

METHIONINE, L-METHIONINE

Methionine is an essential amino acid needed for the synthesis of **protein** in the body. It is a **sulphur-**

containing amino acid and a lipotropic, which means that it has an affinity to fats. As such, it helps to produce **lecithin**, which emulsifies fats and breaks down fatty deposits, preventing their build-up in the liver and arteries and thus reducing the risk of heart and circulatory diseases.

Methionine is a strong detoxifier and combines with toxic elements such as **lead, cadmium** and **mercury** to eliminate them from the body, preventing many related conditions such as hypertension, depression and kidney damage. It is also a strong antioxidant, which neutralizes free radicals, the underlying cause of ageing diseases such as heart disease, cancer and diabetes. Methionine is an anti-histaminic and, as such, can be used in the treatment of allergies. It is best utilized with supplements of **vitamin B6**. Available from health food stores.

MILK

Once promoted as the 'perfect food', cow's milk is an excellent source of **proteins** and **calcium**. Its principal proteins are casein, albumin and globulin. The latter is identical to human blood globulin and, as such, strengthens the immune system by providing antibodies. Milk also provides fat, which aids the absorption of calcium, and its **phosphorus** content offers an ideal calcium–phosphorus ratio, which is required for calcium utilization. In addition, milk contains a good balance of **vitamins A, D, E, K** and **B2** and 1 l of milk a day can supply approximately all the required calcium phosphorus and fat. Milk is a fully digestible food except for those individuals who are unable to digest milk sugar, in a condition known as **lactose intolerance**. However, milk has its drawbacks. It is low in **vitamin C, iron**, and **copper**, and is increasingly considered to be a polluted food in that it may contain residues of pesticides, hormones, DDT, steroids and **antibiotics** (used in udder inflammations). It is also a common allergen and there are many people, including children, who must avoid it. Nevertheless, for most people, milk remains a nourishing food, although many nutritionists now advise that the average daily intake should be less than previously recommended. Organic dairy milk which is preferable, is now becoming increasingly available.

However, for **babies**, cow's milk cannot be considered a good substitute for human milk. Compared to mother's milk, cow's milk is deficient in vitamins A, B1, C and E; its mineral content is three times that of mother's milk and contained in different proportions, and it has more protein and bigger fat globules, which are suited to raising calves but not human babies. The type of lactose in cow's milk (alpha lactose) does not encourage the growth of intestinal flora in babies as does the lactose contained in mother's milk (beta lactose).

Goat's milk is a much more tolerable and suitable form of milk for babies than that of cows. In fact, since the time of Hippocrates, physicians have recommended goat's milk for infants and convalescents because it is so easily digested. Compared to cow's milk, goat's milk has less protein, smaller fat globules, a little more calcium and vitamin A, and nearly 10 times the **fluorine** needed to build strong bones and teeth. Goat's milk is usually given to infants who are allergic to cow's milk or who cannot tolerate the mother's milk. Although goat's milk provides less than 3 per cent of the world milk supply, whole populations in Asia and Africa consume it because 70 per cent of the world's goats are found in those countries.

MILK THISTLE (*Carduus marianus*)

An annual plant that grows wild in dry, rocky soils in parts of Europe and North America, its leaves provide a bitter tonic and its seeds contain flavones (silydanin and silymarin) which stimulates the evacuation of **bile**.

Both the leaves and seeds are used in the treatment of liver diseases and to protect the liver from toxins. Milk thistle is also very beneficial in the treatment of hepatitis and chirrhosis of the liver. And as a general detoxifyer, it can also be useful in the treatment of psoriasis.

In folk medicine, milk thistle was traditionally used to increase milk flow in nursing mothers. It is now widely available in capsules from health food stores or herbalists.

MILLET (*Panicum, Sorghum*)

A small golden pearl grain popular in Asia and Africa, millet is highly nutritious. It is rich in vitamins and minerals, exceptionally high in protein and is the only alkali-forming grain. Millet is rich in **silicon**, which is important for the health of skin, hair and nails. Millet contains no gluten and is therefore suitable for coeliacs. It is very easily digested and useful for diarrhoea, indigestion and diabetes. Millet can be used as a thickener in soups, stews and vegetable casseroles.

MINERALS

Found abundantly on the earth's crust, minerals are essential constituents of all cells. They form mostly the hard parts of the body (bones, teeth, nails), but are equally essential as components of gland secretions and enzyme systems which sustain life. Minerals regulate the permeability of cell membranes, control the excitability of muscles and nerves, maintain a proper acid–alkali balance and regulate blood volume.

Minerals are generally classified into bulk minerals and trace elements. Bulk minerals like **calcium, phosporus, sodium, magnesium, potassium** and **sulphur** are needed in gram amounts. Trace elements, which are needed in minute amounts measured in milligrams or micrograms, include **iron, zinc, copper, manganese, chromium, iodine, selenium, fluorine, boron** and **molybdenum**.

Mineral **salts** are daily used and excreted from the body and must be replaced through food. Minerals are as essential to the body as oxygen; the body can tolerate a deficiency of **vitamins** for longer periods of time than it can a deficiency of minerals. A slight change in the concentration of some minerals in blood can endanger life.

Obviously the mineral content of both plant and animal foods depends entirely on the mineral content of the soil. Different parts of the earth's crust may be deficient in some. The soil of the American Midwest for example, is naturally poor in iodine and in these areas iodized salt is commonly used. On the other hand, intensive farming methods are not always matched by full mineral restoration and this leads to minerally depleted soils and mineral deficiencies in humans. The recent news that selenium levels in English soils have been severely dropping is causing great concern in the UK. On the other hand, the wide consumption of highly refined foods like white sugar and white flour, from which most of the trace elements have been removed during milling, also create mineral shortages. The refining of whole **wheat** to white flour, for example, depletes 80 per cent of its magnesium, 87 per cent of its chromium and 88 per cent of its manganese.

Eating mostly unrefined foods like brown **rice** and wholewheat bread, and cutting down on white sugar, are the first steps towards meeting basic mineral needs.

Minerals are not absorbed as efficiently as **vitamins** Minerals like calcium require a strong acid medium in the stomach to be absorbed, while trace elements require **protein** to enable their absorption into the blood stream (see CHELATION). Mineral supplementation is therefore needed by most people to ensure adequate intake and prevent deficiency symptoms. Special conditions require even higher doses. Iron and calcium, for example, are considered a must for pregnant and lactating women. It is important though not to exceed dosages, as excesses can impair the delicate mineral equilibrium of the body and in extreme cases can even become toxic.

MINT SEE PEPPERMINT

MISO

A savoury fermented **soybean** paste used for seasoning, miso has traditionally been used in China and Japan for many thousands of years. Miso soup is a popular dish in Japanese and Chinese restaurants. Miso is made from cooked soybeans, grain (**barley** or **rice**), **salt** and **water** which are combined with a mould starter. The mixture is then allowed to ferment for between six months and a year.

Miso comes in many varieties and colours and, because it is usually very salty, can be used as a substitute for salt or soy sauce. As a result of fermentation, it is a live food, containing friendly micro-organisms that are beneficial to the intestinal flora. It is therefore best consumed uncooked. Many varieties of miso are available in health food shops.

MISTLETOE (*VISCUM ALBUM*)

An evergreen, semi-parasitic plant which grows on the branches of host trees, it has long been revered as a sacred plant in many European religions and closely associated with magic and healing. Both the leaves and berries are known to be useful in the regulation of high and low blood pressure. Mistletoe has also been used as a nerve tonic in the treatment of tension, insomnia and depression and, prepared as a **tea** from the leaves and berries, it is a diuretic and stimulant and can be used for strengthening the heart. Available at health food stores and herbalists and as formulas.

Caution: Mistletoe is potentially toxic and should not be used in doses greater than 4 g of the crude herb, or for extended periods, except under the supervision of a naturopath.

MOLASSES

Molasses is a concentrated syrup, a by-product of sugar refining, which precipitates as residue after the sugar crystals have been separated from the sugar-cane juice. Molasses is rich in nutrients and low in sugar and, in fact, the nutrients in molasses are 30 times more concentrated than in the original cane juice. It provides an excellent source of **minerals** and trace elements, including **iron, calcium, potassium, magnesium**, copper, **chromium, manganese, molybdenum** and **zinc**. One tablespoon of molasses supplies as much calcium as a glass of **milk** and as much **iron** as nine **eggs**. Molasses also contains high levels of **B vitamins**, and is an alkali-forming food. It is reported to have a beneficial effect on many conditions such as anaemia, fatigue, arthritis, ulcers and colitis. It also has a strong laxative effect and is used to counteract constipation. Unsulphured molasses is better than that preserved with **sulphur**, and crude black molasses is preferable to the sweeter varieties. A normal intake is 1–3 teaspoons a day. Available in health food stores.

Caution: It is recommended that teeth are rinsed after taking molasses because, like sugar, molasses can cause tooth decay.

MOLYBDENUM

Molybdenum is a trace element widely present in raw foods and an essential part of several important **enzymes**. Molybdenum prevents tooth decay and anaemia, and is also thought to prevent oesophageal cancer and increase sexual potency in older men. Since most of the molybdenum content is lost during the milling of whole **grains** and the refining of raw sugar, a diet based on these refined foods can result in a deficiency. The best natural sources of molybdenum are **legumes**, whole grain cereals and dark green leafy vegetables, and a balanced diet should supply adequate amounts of it. The newly set RDA is 45 mcg.

MONOSODIUM GLUTAMATE (MSG)

As a food ingredient, MSG is a flavour enhancer that deserves a special mention since it is commonly used in many processed foods (E621), and especially in Chinese restaurants. An amino acid, MSG is the **sodium salt** of glutamic acid (E620).

MSG was first isolated at the Tokyo University in 1908 from a seaweed (*Laminaria japonica*) which was long known by Japanese cooks to improve food taste. Initially considered safe, MSG was later linked to many allergic symptoms often referred to as 'Chinese Restaurant Syndrome' because they were observed mainly after eating Chinese food. These symptoms include thirst and nausea, water retention, muscle numbness, palpitation, dizziness, headaches and cold sweats.

It should be noted that many foods naturally contain various amounts of glutamate, the highest of which are in **tomatoes**, meatloaves, **mushrooms** and Parmesan cheese. Mother's milk contains 10 times more glutamate than cow's **milk**. But while the body metabolizes food glutamates and MSG in the same way, many people who are allergic to MSG find that they can safely eat glutamate-containing foods like **tomatoes** or **mushrooms**. On average, Americans are considered to consume daily 11 g of glutamate from natural sources and less than 1 g of glutamate from added MSG.

It is estimated that some 25 per cent of the western population is allergic to MSG, in one way or another. Anyone allergic to MSG should realize that, while some food labels may claim 'No MSG', the presence of MSG can be disguised with vague or technical language, such as: glutamic acid; natural flavours; seasoning; modified food starch; autolyzed food yeast.

MSM

A nutritional supplement newly arrived in health food stores, Methylsulphonylmethane, or MSM for simplicity, is a form of organic **sulphur**, the fourth most abundant mineral in the body. A safe, natural and highly assimilable food derived from the ocean, MSM is a white, odourless crystalline powder, which does not produce the intestinal gas or body odour that may occur with other forms of sulphur. The many benefits of sulphur stem from its help in proper cell function, and in creating healthy and flexible cells. MSM supplements are therefore indicated for a variety of reasons such as improving skin, hair and nails, relieving arthritic pain, increasing intestinal fitness and improving conditions like constipation, diarrhoea, overacidity and even food allergies.

Considering the fact that sulphur is a widely deficient mineral that much of it is lost in food preparation, MSM supplementation is becoming increasingly popular. Average daily supplements of MSM range between 1,000 mg and 3,000 mg or more (up to 6,000 mg), depending on body size, age, diet and the nature and severity of the conditions being treated.

Caution: People prone to kidney stones should use MSM cautiously, starting with a low dose. (See SULPHUR.)

MUSHROOMS

Fungi, in the wild, grow most commonly in woods and damp areas; the cultivated varieties are available all-year round. Cultivated mushrooms are one of the most valuable horticultural crops in the UK and the USA. The white *Agaricus bisporus* mushrooms account for over 95 per cent of consumption while speciality or exotic cultivated mushrooms account for the remaining less than 5 per cent. Mushrooms of the button variety are rich in **potassium, phosphorus, copper** and **iron**. They are also a good source of thiamine (**vitamin B1**) and riboflavin (**vitamin B2**). As mushrooms mature, their caps open and expose their gills. It is best to avoid wide open caps and also to select mushrooms that are firm, not spongy.

Mushrooms are known to be beneficial in reducing blood fat levels and to have antibiotic properties; they are also claimed to have anti-tumour actions and to boost the immune system action against disease-producing micro-organisms by increasing white blood cell count.

Mushrooms are easily digested and are recommended for anyone suffering with digestive problems.

MUSTARD (*BRASSICA NIGRA*)

An annual plant native to the temperate regions of the northern hemisphere, it is also widely cultivated for its seeds which contain a strong volatile oil. Mustard is a popular culinary herb that stimulates the **appetite** and helps digestion. A weak **tea** of mustard seeds can be used, in small amounts, for bronchitis or coughs. For external applications, mustard is used mainly as an irritant to promote blood flow in cases of rheumatism and colds.

Mustard seed powder is mixed with wheat flour and water to form a thick paste, and this is then spread on a linen cloth to form a poultice which is laid on the affected area causing the skin to heat up. The poultice must not be used on sensitive areas and it should be removed when the heat becomes too uncomfortable. Wheat flour is added in order to reduce the warming effects of the mustard, and its quantity in the poultice should be adjusted according to the amount of warming desired. Diluted mustard seed oil can also be used externally for similar conditions.

N

NAC (*N-ACETYL CYSTEINE*)

As part of **glutathione**, NAC is a powerful antioxidant and antiviral. It provides protection from free radical damage and strengthens resistance to disease by increasing immune cell levels. As an antioxidant, NAC helps detoxify the liver, prevents cholesterol oxidation, reduces the risk of heart attacks and facilitates the removal of mucous in cystic fibrosis and bronchitis. Available at health food stores.

NADH (*NICOTINAMIDE ADENINE DINUCLEOTIDE*)

A vitamin B3-dependent coenzyme, NADH is essential for cellular energy metabolism and helps produce energy from food. A potent **antioxidant** and stimulant of adrenaline and **dopamine**, NADH is used to relieve chronic fatigue (CFS) and treat Parkinson's and Alzheimer's diseases. Available as a supplement called 'Enada' in health food stores.

NETTLE, STINGING (*URTICA DIOICA*)

Although a coarse herb that grows freely as a weed across Europe, Asia and North America, the leaves, flowers and seeds of the stinging nettle contain a wide range of useful medicinal and culinary properties. The plant makes an effective tonic and can be used to promote **appetite** and eliminate intestinal worms, while its fresh juice will stimulate digestion and promote milk flow in nursing mothers. It is also an astringent and can inhibit urinary tract bleeding, haemorrhoids and excessive menstrual flow. As a decoction, nettle can be used to strengthen the hair and, when used as a wash, to rejuvenate the skin. The leaves of the nettle, which are rich in **vitamins** and **minerals**, are often used to flavour salads and make infusions.

NEUROTRANSMITTERS (*NT*)

Neurotransmitters are special chemicals that carry messages between brain cells. All learning, remembering, sleeping and emotions depend upon the ability of the brain cells to produce and deliver neurotransmitters to other brain cells, as well as to respond to messages from other brain cells.

Neurotransmitters are produced from nutrients absorbed from food. For example, acetylcholine, which is needed by the brain for learning, memory and long-term planning, is made in the body from **choline**, a **B vitamin** found in egg yolk, **grains, legumes**, leafy green vegetables and **lecithin**, which is rich in phosphatidyl choline. Another neurotransmitter, norepinephrine (brain adrenalin), which is needed for wakefulness, sex, learning and body movement, is produced in the brain by **phenylalanine** and **tyrosine**, two **amino acids** that are found in **meat, eggs** and cheese. A deficiency of norepinephrine can cause stress, depression and low sex drive. Other important neurotransmitters include **dopamine, GABA, melatonin** and **serotonin**. Some neurotransmitters, such as norepinephrine, have an excitatory action, while others such as serotonin, have a calming effect.

NIACIN SEE VITAMIN B3

NIGHTSHADES

The nightshades are a class of vegetable that includes
potato, tomatoes, aubergine, peppers and tobacco.
They all contain solanin, a toxic alkaloid that can cause
headaches, osteoarthritis, diarrhoea and vomiting in sensitive
people. Solanine is usually neutralized by cooking, baking,
roasting or frying.

NITRATES, NITRITES

These are chemicals that are used to treat and preserve
bacon and other **meats**, to give them an attractive red
colouring and to prevent botulism and aflatoxin mould.
Nitrates are toxic as they react with **protein** to form
nitrosamines, which are cancer-causing substances. However,
this risk can be reduced by taking supplemental **vitamin C**.

NORI

A seaweed with fibrous, jade-coloured fronds, nori has the
highest protein content of all the **seaweeds** (48 per cent
dry weight) and is also rich in **iodine, sodium, vitamins
A, B1** and niacin. It can help in the treatment of goitre,
and is also used to reduce **cholesterol** levels, alleviate
painful urination, reduce high blood pressure and aid
digestion. It is sold in sheets in health food stores and used
in cooking.

Nori is best known for its use in the preparation of sushi.

NUCLEIC ACIDS

Nucleic acids are special **proteins** that contain the genetic code and heredity information for the human body. They are present in all cells and supervise their growth, multiplication and functioning. They consist of DNA (deoxyribonucleic acid), which contains the master 'blueprint', and RNA (ribonucleic acid), which acts as the messenger to the cells. Nucleic acids are vulnerable to free radical damage in that free radicals oxidize the nucleic acids and cross-link their molecules, distorting their information. This distorted information can lead to mutations in cell multiplication and performance, cancer and premature ageing. DNA and RNA can be protected by **antioxidant vitamins** and nutrients. Nucleic acids are available as nutritional supplements.

Caution: Nucleic acid supplements are not suitable for people with gout as they increase uric acid levels.

NUTMEG (*MYRISTICA FRAGRANS*)

A tropical evergreen tree native to the Molucca (Spice) Islands, it is now cultivated in Indonesia, the West Indies, Brazil, India and Sri Lanka for its aromatic seeds which are used mainly as a culinary spice, also known as mace. The ground seeds improve **appetite**, stimulate digestion and relieve flatulence. It is also a mild hallucinogenic.

Caution: Eating nutmeg in more than seasoning amounts can be dangerous. Overdoses can produce poisoning symptoms such as stomach pain, dizziness and delirium. Widely available ground or whole in supermarkets.

OATS (*AVENA SATIVA*)

Oats are an exceptional cereal and are used primarily for their outstanding nutritional value. They are a few times higher in **protein** and fat content than any other cereal and are also rich in **vitamin E**, some of the **B vitamins** and **minerals**, particularly **zinc, manganese** and silica. They are high in **fibre** and, prepared as a porridge, can help to prevent constipation, soothe the digestive system, reduce **cholesterol** and strengthen the heart. They are also useful in conditions such as weakness, diabetes, hepatitis, indigestion and bloating. Oats help to strengthen bones as they are rich in silica, and a tincture of oats has been reported to reduce cravings for cigarettes. In addition to porridge, oats are also used in soups, puddings, breads and desserts. Although oats do not contain gluten, the issue of oats for coeliacs is not entirely clear.

OCTACOSANOL

An ingredient of **wheat germ oil**, it has been found to increase energy, endurance and strength by increasing oxygen utilization in muscles during **exercise**. Octacosanol also benefits muscular dystrophy and other nerve–muscle disorders. It is available on its own or incorporated into nutritional formulas (see WHEAT GERM OIL).

OLIVE OIL

One of the most desirable culinary oils, especially when it is extra virgin, cold pressed and unrefined, the main fatty acid in olive oil, oleic acid, is a monounsaturated, omega-9 fatty acid. Being monounsaturated, olive oil is more stable, less vulnerable to rancidity and more resistant to heat than polyunsaturated oils such as safflower, sunflower and **corn**. It is therefore highly recommended for cooking. Olive oil is also excellent used fresh in salad dressings, and is a popular folk remedy in Mediterranean countries for gallstones; it is also claimed to help flush out kidney stones, particularly when a tablespoon of olive oil is taken following fresh **lemon** juice made of two medium-size lemons. Olive oil is also used for constipation and its continuous use is well-known to help lower high **cholesterol** levels. Externally, olive oil can be used to treat burns, bruises and sprains.

OLIVE TREE LEAVES

A food and medicine since biblical times, olive leaves have now been 'rediscovered' as an energizing food with antiviral and antibacterial properties. As far back as 1855, information started to spread that drinking bitter **tea** brewed from olive tree leaves was a potential cure for malaria. More recently, the active ingredients in the leaves, two phenolic compounds (oleuropein and elenolate), have been isolated. Oleuropein has been found to inhibit two types of fermentative bacteria – which, incidentally, is why olives are often cracked before pickling and the phenols removed, since they inhibit fermentation.

Olive leaf extract is increasingly used as a supplement to treat chronic fatigue and boost the immune system. It is also recommended for sore throats, coughs and sinus problems. Oleuropein has been found to be an effective antioxidant, preventing **cholesterol** from oxidization. As such, it is used to reduce the risk of coronary heart disease in vulnerable people, since oxidized cholesterol is easily deposited, causing blocked blood vessels. Olive leaf extract is now available in capsule form from the Allergy Research Group in San Leandro CA, USA.

OMEGA-3 FATTY ACIDS

These are types of essential, polyunsaturated fatty acids. They include EPA (eicosapentaenoic acid) and DHA (docosahexaenoic acid) which are found mainly in ocean fish like **salmon**, mackerel and sardines, and ALA (alphalinolenic acid) found mainly in **flaxseed** oil. The omega-3 fatty acids are very important to the body's health. They reduce blood stickiness, **blood clotting, cholesterol** levels, blood pressure and inflammations. In this way they help to prevent heart attacks and strokes. In one study, a daily consumption of 1–5 g of omega-3 fatty acids was found to reduce the death risk of coronary heart disease in men by 40 per cent. Supplemental EPA was shown to reduce the levels of triglycerides and fibrinogen, a **protein** involved in blood clotting.

ALA can be converted in the body to EPA and, similarly, EPA can be converted to DHA. EPA however, is considered the most beneficial of the omegas. It is the best source for the body's own production of beneficial prostaglandins that also help reduce inflammation. As such, EPA is considered very helpful in heart disease and inflammatory conditions like arthritis, and is the reason why heart patients and arthritics are often advised to eat ocean **fish** instead of **meat**. EPA is now also available in capsule form, and is sold as a food supplement in health food stores. DHA is particularly important for the eye tissue and for brain development in infancy.

OMEGA-6 FATTY ACIDS

Omega-6 is a group of several essential fatty acids, most notably, Linoleic acid (LA) and **Arachidonic Acid (AA)**. They are mostly abundant in cooking oils, especially in soybean oil, corn oil and sunflower oil, and in everyday foods like poultry, eggs, avocado, nuts and cereals.

Although Omega-6, like Omega-3, is an essential polyunsaturated fatty acid, involved in many biological processes such as blood clotting and inflammation, they act in opposite ways. While Omega-6 fatty acids tend to promote inflammatory conditions (in response to infections and injuries), Omega-3 fatty acids have an anti-inflammatory effect. A proper balance between the two is thus important. An intake ratio of four parts Omega-6 to one part Omega-3 which is considered ideal, was found in primitive societies which have thrived in good health throughout history, such as the Inuits. The problem is that Omega-6 is prevalent in most of today's foods, which is why we consume Omega-6 in excessive amounts, compared to Omega-3 foods, in ratios of 14: 1 in the best case, up to 30:1 in the worst case. This imblance increases inflammatory conditions. And that is one of the reasons why the degenerative afflictions of civilisation such as heart disease, arthritis, stroke and cancer are so widespread. To balance our ratios, we can cut down the use of the highest sources of Omega-6 such as soybean oil, and use instead lower sources of Omega-6 like **olive oil** and coconut oil. Alternatively, we can eat more seafood like salmon, sardines and mackerel, and take supplements such as **linseed oil**, **cod liver oil** or **Omega-3** capsules which can improve the ratio of our Omegas even further.

ONION (*ALLIUM*)

Probably first grown in central or south-western Asia, nowadays onions are grown throughout the world, mainly for their culinary properties, although for many centuries they have been recognized also for their medicinal value. The healing properties of onions are now scientifically established and are attributed to their many important components, such as **quercetin, mustard** oils andsulphur-containing compounds. Onions can reduce blood stickiness, preventing blood clots and heart attacks. Crude extracts of onion have been shown to lower high blood pressure and **cholesterol** levels. Onions are also used to expel phlegm and alleviate coughs, colds and inflammations of the nose and throat. Onion soup can help cure hangovers and is good for coughs, colds and bronchitis.

ORANGE (*CITRUS SINENSIS*)

The orange is among the oldest known cultivated fruits and has been grown for more than 4,000 years. It probably originated in the south-western regions of Asia, but nowadays is cultivated in subtropical climates worldwide.

Orange is an acidic fruit, best known for its high **vitamin C** content – 60 mg per 100 g edible fruit – which is always highest in the early part of the season and much lower in the late season. Oranges also contain **vitamin A, potassium, calcium, phosphorus** and **folic acid**. The white part of the rind is a rich source of **pectin**, which lowers **cholesterol**, and of **bioflavonoids**, which benefits weak gums, capillaries and blood vessels. In fact, sweetened orange peel is a popular Middle Eastern treat. The fruit itself has strong anti-inflammatory effects and can be used as a general tonic; it improves digestion and is beneficial for conditions such as colds, arthritis and fevers. The oil derived from the orange rind can relieve flatulence.

OREGANO (*ORIGANUM VULGARE*)

A perennial herb, native to the Mediterranean regions, oregano is commonly used as a culinary herb. Infusions of the leaves, flowers and stalks can benefit an upset stomach, colic, headaches, nervousness, coughs, whooping cough and other respiratory disorders. Oregano also promotes perspiration, relieves flatulence and expels phlegm. Oregano **tea** can be used to relieve abdominal cramps in women and regulate the menstrual cycle when taken three or four days before the period is due.

   Caution: Oregano should not be used during pregnancy.

ORNITHINE, L-ORNITHINE

Ornithine is derived from **arginine**, and shares its properties in that it is a **growth-hormone** releaser and strengthens the immune system. However, supplemental ornithine should be taken in half the quantities recommended for arginine.

OXALIC ACID

Oxalic acid is a nutrient found in various vegetables and fruits, particularly in **spinach, rhubarb**, beets and cranberries;

it is also found in **chocolate**. Consumption of oxalic acid-containing foods can increase any tendency to kidney stones or gravel since the oxalic acid in the food may combine with **calcium**, resulting in calcium-oxalate kidney stones. People with a known tendency to kidney stones or gravel would therefore do well to cut down on the amount of oxalic acid-containing foods in their diet.

OKRA (*ABELMOSCHUS ESCULENTUS*)

A native of Africa, okra – also known as gumbo, ladies' fingers or bamia – is grown in large quantities in the southern states of the USA. It is also very popular in Middle Eastern cooking. An annual, the vegetable is produced for its green pods which contain large amounts of **vitamins A** and **C, calcium, phosphorus, potassium** and **magnesium**. Okra is the number one vegetable source of **manganese**. The plant is also rich in mucilaginous substances, which lubricate the intestines and are recommended for soothing duodenal ulcers and reducing high **cholesterol** levels.

OYSTERS

Found mainly in oceans and coastal regions with mild to tropical climates, oysters are one of the richest sources of **zinc** and are often recommended as an aphrodisiac to increase fertility and sex drive. Fresh oysters contain 149 mg zinc per 100 g of the edible portions. The shell is a rich source of **calcium** and is sometimes used in calcium supplements.

Caution: Because of their **zinc** content, oysters should be eaten only in moderation.

P

PABA (*PARA AMINO BENZOIC ACID*)

An **antioxidant** vitamin related to **folic acid**, PABA is
the 'sun screen' vitamin that protects the skin from
sunburn. It is known for its ability to absorb ultraviolet
(UV) light, thus preventing wrinkling of the skin and
reducing the risk of skin cancer. It is therefore widely used
in sunblock preparations.

PABA also has other beneficial effects. It corrects loss
of pigmentation in skin and hair, prevents hair greying and
retards hair loss. It also protects the lungs from ozone
damage, acts as a **coenzyme** in the utilization of **protein**
and assists the formation of red blood cells.

Deficiency symptoms include skin conditions such as
eczema and wrinkles, fatigue, irritability and depression,
senility, arthritis and bursitis. Among its best natural sources
are organ **meats, brewer's yeast**, whole **grains**, raw
wheat germ and **molasses**. No Recommended Daily
Allowances have been established, but an allowance of
between 30 mg and 100 mg is considered reasonable. In
spite of the fact that the body synthesizes PABA, it may
not be sufficient for maximum protection and therefore
PABA supplements can usefully enhance its beneficial
effects.

PANCREATIN

This is the name given to digestive-aid tablets containing pancreatic **enzymes** such as protease, lipase and amylase. These enzymes break down **proteins, fats** and starch, and assist in their digestion. Pancreatin tablets can prevent bloating, stomach discomfort, indigestion and gastroenteritis (inflammation of the stomach and intestines), and are normally taken after main meals to strengthen digestion.

Since the secretion of digestive enzymes is reduced with age, pancreatin tablets are often recommended by some nutritionists even for healthy people over 40. Pancreatin can also prevent food allergies that arise from by-products of incomplete digestion.

PANGAMIC ACID

Pangamic acid, or vitamin B15, is used mainly in Russia to improve heart conditions and athletic performance. It is still not fully officially accepted in the west. It is an antioxidant and prevents the formation of destructive superoxide radicals, a major cause of ageing. It is also an antipollutant, eliminating environmental toxins from the body. Being a lipotropic substance, it lowers **cholesterol** levels and prevents fat accumulation in the liver. A lack of pangamic acid can cause reduced oxygenation of the blood, leading to fatigue and lowered fitness. Its best natural sources are **brewer's yeast**, brown rice, whole **grains, pumpkin** and **sesame seeds**. There are no

Recommended Daily Allowances, but a daily intake of 25–100 mg is normal. It is sometimes available as a supplement called 'calcium pangamate'.

PANTOTHENIC ACID

Although pantothenic acid, also called **vitamin B5**, occurs in small amounts in most foods, a deficiency of the vitamin is commonplace. It is involved in a number of metabolic functions, such as fat and sugar metabolism and the production of adrenalin, which is needed in stress conditions. It also helps to maintain normal **blood sugar** levels and increase energy, particularly in stressful situations – which is why it is often called the 'stress vitamin'. It is also used to treat rheumatoid arthritis and allergies. Pantothenic acid is an important ingredient of **royal jelly** and cod's roe, hence its use for improving fertility and reproduction.

Some indications of a deficiency of the vitamin include stress, irritability or depression, low blood sugar levels, fatigue, indigestion, constipation, ulcers, arthritis and allergies. Among the best natural sources are royal jelly, cod's roe, **brewer's yeast**, organ **meats**, raw wheat germ, whole **grains**, beans, **molasses** and nuts.

The Recommended Daily Allowance for pantothenic acid is set at 10 mg, but most nutritionists recommend 30–50 mg a day. It is available as a supplement on its own, and is also included in B complex and multivitamin supplements.

PAPAIN SEE PAPAYA

PAPAYA, PAWPAW, PAPAIN (*CARICA PAPAYA*)

A sweet tropical fruit, which is eaten fresh and is best known for its ability to aid digestion. Papaya contains the enzyme papain which helps to digest **proteins** and is therefore useful for the relief of dyspepsia and weak digestion. It is also helpful in cases of food allergies caused by incomplete digestion of **protein** fragments. In tropical regions, papaya has long been used as a **meat** tenderizer, and it is also known to expel worms, treat dysentery and relieve rheumatic pain. Papaya is a rich source of **beta carotene** (provitamin A) and **vitamins B** and **C**, making it a very nutritious food. It is increasingly used in the manufacture of commercial digestive aids and skin creams.

PARSLEY (*Petroselinum crispum*)

Parsley is a very popular biennial herb with aromatic leaves that are used as a culinary flavouring. The leaves are either eaten fresh in salads or steeped for **tea**. Parsley is an excellent diuretic and is useful for kidney disorders and the elimination of stones and gravel. Both the fresh juice and a tea made from the leaves or seeds can be used to relieve water retention (oedema) and strengthen digestion. Parsley also stimulates delayed menstruation and promotes menstrual flow.

PARSNIP (*Pastinaca sativa*)

A sweet culinary root vegetable and mildly diuretic, it lubricates the intestines and is beneficial for soothing stomach and intestinal irritations. It helps to clean the liver and gall bladder and, used in soups or **teas**, it promotes perspiration and is beneficial for coughs, colds, headaches and arthritis.

Caution: Only the root part of the plant should be eaten. Parsnip leaves are poisonous.

PASSION FLOWER (*PASSIFLORA INCARNATA*)

A strong climbing vine which grows wild and is also cultivated as a garden plant, the flowers are used mainly to calm nervousness and hysteria, relieve headaches and induce sleep. A **tea** (available from health food stores) prepared from the flowers is effective against involuntary cramps and for high blood pressure caused by nervous conditions. The fruit is sold as a delicacy in some shops and can be used for conserving and flavouring.

PAU D'ARCO (*TABEVULIA*)

A South American bitter herb which is antibacterial, antifungal and a booster of the immune system. It has traditionally been used to control candida (thrush) and help in the treatment of cancer. It is also used to cleanse the blood, treat liver disease, infections, diabetes, ulcers, allergies and tumours. Pau d'arco is available as tea bags in many health food shops.

PAWPAW SEE PAPAYA

PEAS (*PISUM SATIVUM*)

Native to temperate climates, fresh peas are sweet and juicy, and one of the most digestible and non-gassy **legumes**. They contain 78 per cent **water**, with only traces of fat, are low in **sodium** and provide a good source of **iron** and **vitamins A, C, B1, B2** and niacin. Peas have a diuretic and mildly laxative effect and are recommended for strengthening digestion, reducing water retention and helping to promote elimination. They are popular as a summer vegetable and also make a nutritious addition to salads, soups and casseroles.

PEACH (*PRUNUS PERSICA*)

A deciduous tree, grown in temperate climates, it is believed that the peach was originally native to China where it has been grown for several thousand years. It was spread throughout Europe by the Romans and first taken to North America in the sixteenth century by the Spanish explorers. Peaches are a delicious fruit, providing a rich source of **beta carotene, iron** and **calcium**, together with some **vitamin C** and niacin. The fruit is astringent and tends to limit perspiration. It can also be used to alleviate coughs and gastrointestinal inflammations.

PEANUTS (*ARACHIS HYPOGAEA*)

A legume that is now grown throughout the warm regions of the world, particularly in Africa and Asia, the peanut was originally native to South America. Peanuts are high in fat and rich in **protein**, niacin, **calcium** and **magnesium**. Due to their high oil content, they are best eaten raw or lightly roasted and, since they contain almost 49 per cent fat, they are not very suitable for dieters. Peanuts lubricate the intestines and are useful for the alleviation of ulcers or digestive tract tumours. They are known to increase milk flow in nursing mothers, to curb internal bleeding and improve hearing. A tea made from the shells was traditionally used to lower high blood pressure. Eaten in moderation, peanuts can benefit underweight people.

Caution: Large amounts can cause skin problems. Peanuts are a heavily sprayed nut and are subject to aflatoxin, a carcinogenic fungus. It is safer, therefore, to eat organically grown peanuts.

PEAR (*PYRUS COMMUNIS*)

Closely related to the **apple** and the quince, pears are grown throughout the temperate regions of the world. The fruit is high in **water** and **fibre** but low in **vitamin C** and **minerals**. Pears can be used to alleviate constipation, coughs and sore throats; the **fibre** will soothe intestinal inflammations.

Caution: Excessive use of pears is not recommended, especially during pregnancy, since their **fibre** taxes digestion.

PECAN (*CARYA*)

Native to North America, the tree is grown throughout the southern states of the USA and, to a lesser extent, in South Africa, Australia and the Middle East. It is valued for its fruit, the pecan nut, which is rich in fat and provides one of the highest sources of unsaturated fatty acids. About 75 per cent of its total **calories** come from its fat content. The pecan nut is therefore very calorific and although, nutritionally, it is high in **potassium** and **B vitamins**, it contains far too many calories for the amount of **protein** it provides. Pecans are delicious and best eaten fresh before their oils become rancid but, due to their high calorific value, they are not very suitable for anyone who is overweight or on a weight-reducing diet.

PECTIN

Pectin is a gel-forming dietary **fibre** that forms part of plant cells and is found mainly in the skins, peels and rinds of fruits and vegetables. **Orange** rind contains 30 per cent pectin, **apple** peel 15 per cent and **onion** skin 12 per cent. Pectin has several nutritional roles: it binds **cholesterol** and **bile** acids in the intestines, promoting their excretion and thus helping to lower high cholesterol levels; pectin also binds with toxic metals such as **lead, mercury** and **cadmium**, and with radioactive residues, and excretes them from the body. Pectin supplements sold in health food stores have been found to be helpful in controlling diabetes, treating constipation and reducing the risk of heart attacks. Pectin is also used as a stabilizer and thickener (E440b) in commercially processed jams and preserves.

PEPPERS (*CAPSICUM*)

Originating in South America and brought to Europe in the sixteenth century, the pepper is now grown throughout much of the world – as a perennial in tropical regions and, in temperate areas, as an annual. Its colourful fruit – red, green and yellow peppers, or capsicums – provide an excellent source of **beta carotene** and **vitamin C**; they also contain high amounts of **calcium, phosphorus, sodium** and **potassium**. Peppers also contain two other important **carotenoids**, lutein and zeaxanthin, both of which can help protect against age-related macular degeneration (AMD), which can lead to a loss of central vision in the elderly. Peppers can improve **appetite** and digestion, promote circulation and reduce swellings.

Caution: Peppers are a known allergen that can cause reactions in many people. If an allergy is suspected, it is best to avoid peppers for a week, then try them again to check for any recurrence of symptoms. Usually, people allergic to raw peppers will find they can safely eat them if cooked.

PEPPERMINT, MINT (*MENTHA*)

A perennial herb of the mint family, which grows best in moist soils, it is widely cultivated in the temperate regions of Europe and North America. The herb contains menthol and is popular as both a flavouring agent and a **tea**. It is also well known for its carminative effects – that is, it helps to relieve flatulence and indigestion. Since menthol is also an **appetite** stimulant, digestive and sedative, peppermint can be used to prevent or alleviate cramps, insomnia and vomiting; it is also claimed to be an aphrodisiac. In addition, peppermint has antiviral properties: its tannins have been found to suppress the activity of the flu virus and inhibit Herpes simplex. Peppermint oil is used to relieve the symptoms of irritable bowel syndrome (IBS).

PERSIMMON (*DIOSPYROS VIRGINIANA*)

A small tree that belongs to the ebony family, two of its species are grown for their pulpy, edible fruits. One of these, the kaki or Japanese persimmon, is native to central and northern China, while the other, the common persimmon, is native to the south-eastern United States.

Ripe persimmons are sweet fruits that soothe the digestive tract and help to relieve gastro-intestinal inflammations such as enteritis. Persimmons contain diospyrol, an active ingredient found effective against parasitic infections, and in Thailand the fruit is used to expel worms. Unripe persimmons contain tannins and are astringent, which makes them beneficial in treating diarrhoea, dysentery, hypertension and coughs. However, it is important not to eat them in large quantities, certainly not more than one or two at a time, as it is known to cause intestinal blockage in some people.

PHENYLALANINE (PA), L-PHENYLALANINE

An essential amino acid that is abundant in **meat** and cheese, and without which the body cannot synthesize **protein**, PA has many important roles. It helps to form insulin, a hormone controlling **blood sugar** levels, and it is a precursor of **tyrosine**, which is needed by the thyroid gland to produce its hormone, thyroxine. PA is converted in the brain to epinephrine and norepinephrine, excitatory types of brain adrenalines which promote mental alertness, alleviate depression and suppress **appetite** very effectively, thus assisting in weight loss.

PA comes in two forms, L-phenylalanine (LPA) and D-phenylalanine (DPA), which are mirror images of each other: LPA has the nutritional value, while DPA has painkilling and depression-alleviating properties. A third form, DL-phenylalanine (DLPA) is both nutritional and therapeutic.

Studies have shown that DLPA can alleviate the pains of chronic conditions such as arthritis, lower back pain and headaches by protecting endorphins – the natural pain-blocking hormones secreted by the nerve cells. Available at health food stores.

Caution: Excessive doses of phenylalanine or DLPA can cause irritability, insomnia and elevated blood pressure.

People with hypertension would do best to consult a nutritionist before taking DLPA. They should be started on a low dose (100 mg daily), which is then gradually increased while, at the same time, a check is kept on their blood pressure which should be monitored frequently.

PHOSPHATIDYLSERINE (PS)

Phosphatidylserine is a relatively recently discovered nutrient that is normally produced by the brain. However, deficiencies of certain nutrients such as **folic acid**, **vitamin B12** and essential fatty acid can inhibit its production. PS is a vital phospholipid that maintains the integrity of brain cells, and its supplementation has been found to improve mental function by increasing the levels of acetylcholine, which transmits brain messages. However, its primary use is in the treatment of memory loss, depression, and behavioural and age-related brain changes in the elderly.

Phosphatidylserine supplements, which are available in formulas in combination with other brain-enhancing nutrients, are becoming increasingly popular in health food shops.

PHOSPHORUS

Phosphorus is the second most abundant mineral in the body. It co-operates with **calcium** to ensure good bone mineralization and is present in every cell of the body. It is a constituent of DNA, the holder of our genetic blueprint, and of myelin, which insulates nerves. It is vital for the release of energy, converting **glucose** to glycogen (stored sugar) and helping to form **lecithin**. Phosphorus maintains strong bones and teeth, promotes growth and body repair, provides energy by helping to metabolize **carbohydrates** and **fats**, ensures proper functioning of nerves and maintains an acid–alkaline balance.

Phosphorus deficiencies are rare, but the mineral can be depleted by sugar and **antacids**, and deficiency symptoms include weak bones and teeth, rickets, gum infections, arthritis, loss of **appetite** and muscle weakness. Its best natural sources include **meat, eggs, fish**, whole **grains**, raw wheat germ, nuts and seeds. The normal daily requirement for adults is 800 mg, and for lactating women 1,200 mg.

PHYTIC ACID

Phytic acid, or inositol hexaphosphate, is a form of **inositol**, one of the **B vitamins**. A component of the **bran** contained in **grains**, seeds and **legumes**, phytic acid binds with **calcium, magnesium, iron, zinc** and other **minerals**, preventing their absorption in the body. Thus, in order to prevent mineral deficiencies, it must be deactivated, and this can be done by bread-leavening, baking, or seed-sprouting.

Caution: Consumption of large quantities of raw bran can result in a deficiency of minerals such as calcium unless supplements of multi-mineral tablets are taken.

PINEAPPLES (*ANANAS*)

Although pineapples are a rich source of **vitamin C** and **potassium**, they are low in other nutrients. However, they contain **bromelain**, a **protein**-splitting enzyme which increases digestion ability, and they can therefore be usefully eaten after a **meat** dish. **Bromelain** is also sold in capsules as a supplemental digestive aid. Pineapples are also diuretic and can be used to increase **appetite**, strengthen digestion, treat diarrhoea, destroy worms and reduce oedema.

Caution: Since unripe pineapples are acidic, they should not be eaten by anyone with a stomach or duodenal ulcer. Their acidity can also damage teeth.

PISTACHIO NUTS

Originating from the Middle East, pistachios are a popular snack for their high nutritional value and potential health benefits. Pistachios are high in protein (20 per cent), rich in fibre (10 per cent) and a good source of minerals, especially **potassium**, **copper** and **iron**. They contain several B vitamins, particularly **B1** and **B6**, **vitamin E**, **carotenoids** and polyphenolic antioxidant compounds which protect body cells from the oxidative damage of free radicals. Their high fat content of 45 per cent is mostly mono and unsaturated fatty acids, which help improve blood lipid's profile. Even though 100 g pistachios provide 557 calories, they don't promote weight gain due to their high satiety effect. In Middle Eastern countries pistachios are reputed to be aphrodisiacs. And indeed, pistachios were found to be high in **arginine**, an amino acid which raises levels of nitric oxide, a compound that increases blood flow and promotes penile erection. Pistachios are best eaten raw rather than roastd.

PLUMS, PRUNES (*PRUNUS*)

Grown mainly in the temperate regions of the northern hemisphere, plums are high in **potassium**, and also contain moderate levels of **calcium** and **iron**. Due to their low fat content, they are a low-calorie food, and some of the golden varieties are a good source of **beta carotene**. Plums are diuretic and can be used in the treatment of liver conditions such as cirrhosis. Prunes are the dried fruit of a sweet variety of plum which is much richer in sugars, calcium and iron than standard plums. They contain a substance (dihydroxyphenyl isatin) which stimulates the bowels. Stewed prunes, or prune juice, have a laxative effect and are a traditional remedy for constipation.

POMEGRANATE (*PUNICA GRANATUM*)

The fruit of a plant native to the warm climates of India and the Middle East, pomegranates have a potent anti-oxidant activity due to their punicalagins, which are valuable in the maintenance of a healthy cardiovascular system. Pomegranates are a sweet-and-sour fruit, rich in **iron** and astringent. They are used to control diarrhoea and expel intestinal worms, but can also be helpful for treating bladder disturbances, strengthening gums and soothing mouth ulcers.

POPPY (*PAPAVER SOMNIFERUM*)

An annual herb, which is found wild in Asia and across Europe, it is noted for its brilliant red flowers. Although the seeds and oil of the plant have traditionally been used in cooking – particularly in bread and cake-making – the acutely poisonous nature of the seeds should not be dismissed. When the unripe seed pods are crushed, they yield a milky juice that quickly hardens – and this is opium. Opium contains 25 different alkaloids, most of which are highly addictive; these include morphine, the well-known pain-reliever, codeine and heroin.

Caution: Both the plant and its derivatives are poisonous and should be used only on prescription.

POTASSIUM

Potassium is a bulk mineral which constitutes 5 per cent of the total mineral content of the body. It is found mainly in intracellular fluids (i.e. fluids within cells), and has a multitude of functions. Together with **sodium**, potassium regulates the sodium-potassium balance that affects water retention and stimulates kidney function; it also promotes insulin secretion and is involved in nerve transmission and muscle contraction. In addition, potassium promotes the disposal of the body's wastes, enhances mental alertness by increasing oxygen supply to the brain, reduces blood pressure, benefits diabetics by stimulating insulin production and helps digestion by stimulating stomach secretions.

Potassium deficiency symptoms include water retention (oedema), hypertension, irregular heartbeat, nervousness, fatigue and arthritis. Among the best natural sources of the mineral are citrus fruits, leafy green vegetables, bananas, **potato, tomatoes** and **pineapples**. Potassium deficiencies are rare, but can occur in cases of excessive diarrhoea or vomiting, or in the prolonged use of diuretics. In such cases, potassium supplements are necessary, and they are also sometimes recommended for diabetics to improve their insulin sensitivity. No daily requirements are set for potassium, but an average daily consumption for adults of 1.9–5.6 g is considered normal.

POTATO (*SOLANUM TUBEROSUM*)

A member of the nightshade family, *Solanaceae*, the potato is a native of South America and was first introduced into Europe in the mid-sixteenth century. Nowadays, it is the world's most widely grown vegetable and one of its most important foods. Potatoes have a high nutritional value and are grown in most countries. They are a highly starchy food and, when eaten with the skin or peel, a good source of vegetable **protein, potassium, vitamin C, iron, phosphorus**, niacin and **enzymes** – although old potatoes are low in **vitamin C**. Medicinally, potatoes can help to relieve arthritis and reduce water retention due to their high potassium content. They also neutralize body acids, and potato juice can be used to treat stomach and duodenal ulcers. The fresh juice is sometimes used to reduce hypertension and promote intestinal flora.

Potatoes are a member of the solanum family which contains poisonous solanine. Potatoes that develop green skin colouring after flowering are poisonous because of an accumulation of solanine, and can cause indigestion or affect the nervous system. The plant leaves are totally indigestible.

PREGNENOLONE

A recently highlighted natural hormone (also known as preg), it is formed from **cholesterol** in the organs that produce steroid hormones, such as the adrenal glands, and is a precursor of **DHEA**. Apart from its conversion to **DHEA** or progesterone, preg has also been claimed to improve energy, enhance mental acuity, regulate mood disorders and relieve fatigue. In addition, it is reputed to improve memory and learning capabilities. It is currently used mainly for its benefits in chronic conditions such as arthritis, psoriasis and pre-menstrual syndrome. However, although pregnenolone is now being sold over the counter in the USA, it should be used with caution since, to date, relatively little research has been done on it.

PRESERVATIVES

Preservatives are additives, usually chemicals such as **nitrates** and phosphates, that are added during the processing of food to prevent spoilage and reduce food– poisoning risks by inhibiting the growth of bacteria, viruses and fungi. Nowadays, a wide range of foods are commercially preserved, from soft drinks, jams and cheeses to **beer, wine** and **meats**. Some of the most popular preservatives, such as **benzoic acid**, benzoates, **sulphur** dioxide and particularly sulphites have been reported to trigger allergic reactions such as asthma in susceptible people.

PROANTHOCYANIDINS SEE BIOFLAVONOIDS

PROBIOTICS

This is a general descriptive name for all products that regenerate the intestines and rejuvenate the whole body. Probiotics enhance the growth of intestinal flora – the friendly bacteria in the intestines – while reducing disease-causing bacteria. In general, they promote healthy biological systems, as opposed to **antibiotics** and the contraceptive pill which do the opposite, promoting decaying processes in the gut. Probiotics include **yogurts**, buttermilk and other sour milks, digestive **enzymes, FOS** and fermented foods such as **sauerkraut, miso** and **tofu**. Yogurts and sour milks contain cultures of friendly bacteria, including *Lactobacillus acidophilus*, *Lactobacillus bulgaricus, Bifidobacteria longum and Streptococcus thermophilus*, which are usually listed on the food labels.

When consumed regularly, these friendly bacteria are highly beneficial to the body. They assist food absorption, increase the production of **vitamins**, maintain proper acidity in the intestines, increase resistance against disease and prevent the development of colon cancer and thrush (candida). **FOS** are types of sugars that feed selectively only the friendly bacteria and enhance their growth. Overgrowth of pathogenic bacteria in the intestines is associated with conditions such as allergies, eczema, bad breath, constipation, arthritis, headaches, sinus congestion, high **cholesterol**, colitis, candida, yeast infections and cystitis.

PROLINE, L-PROLINE

One of the non-essential **amino acids**, proline supplements are recommended in the treatment of short- term depression. They are claimed to give many people a sense of relief and happiness. Proline is also involved in the production of collagen and can therefore improve skin texture. Available at health food stores and as formulas.

PROPOLIS

Hailed as a natural antibiotic, propolis is a resinous substance collected by bees from plants and trees. Propolis is composed mostly of resins, balsams and waxes, and partly of pollen and essential oils, which are all mixed by the bees' salivary glands and used in the construction of the hive. It has been used throughout history for a wide range of conditions and its name, pro-polis, which signifies its protective effects, comes from the Greek, meaning 'defence before the city'.

Propolis contains a great variety of **amino acids,
vitamins, minerals** and **bioflavonoids** and, in the same
way that it is used by the bees as a sticky filler to seal,
protect and sterilize the hive, propolis can be used for similar
beneficial effects on the human body. For instance, the Greeks
used it to treat wounds and Hippocrates himself, the father of
modern medicine, prescribed propolis for sores and ulcers.

During the past twenty years, scientific studies have
'rediscovered' propolis and found it to be a great booster
of the immune system, enhancing the immune response
and resistance against disease by stimulating the formation
of immune cells. A recent study at Oxford University has
revealed that propolis can help to cure inflammations, while
Chinese research has found propolis effective in treating
hypertension and arteriosclerosis, and Russian scientists have
shown that propolis can prevent ulcers.

Having a potent antibacterial and antifungal action,
propolis is now increasingly used to treat conditions as
wide-ranging as colds, sore throats, coughs, allergies, vaginal
infections, painful menstruation, acne and herpes.

When buying propolis it is important to check on the
quantity in each capsule. The recommended dosage is 1.5–3
g per day, which should be taken on an empty stomach,
preferably first thing in the morning or at bedtime. The
main flavonoid ingredients required to identify it as genuine
propolis are galanagin, chrysin and pinocembrin.

PROSTAGLANDINS SEE EVENING PRIMROSE OIL (EPO); FATS

PROTEIN

As a macronutrient, protein is the most plentiful component of the body, after **water**. It not only builds up body structures such as cells, tissues and skeleton, but also creates the body's functional factors, such as hormones, antibodies, DNA and digestive secretions. Protein enables children's growth, and is equally important in adulthood, when growth has ceased, to supply 'spare parts' to counteract the wear and tear of daily living. Various proteins, such as those in red blood cells, hormones and immune cells, are constantly being broken down and need to be rebuilt. Proteins also serve as a source of energy and heat, providing 4 **calories** per g. Their richest dietary sources are animal foods such as **eggs, meat, fish** and dairy products.

Protein is made up of **amino acids**, in the same way that a wall is composed of bricks, and during the digestion process it is broken down in the body to its basic 'bricks', the amino acids, which are then absorbed into the bloodstream and reassembled for new protein synthesis. Twenty-two amino acids are linked together in various forms to create the many and varied types of proteins, such as hair, bone or nails, and these processes are supervised by the **nucleic acids** RNA and DNA, the specific proteins that contain our genetic blueprint. Eight of these amino acids, which cannot be produced by the body and must be supplied by food, are classified as 'essential amino acids', namely: **leucine, isoleucine, valine**, methionine, **threonine, lysine, phenylalanine** and **tryptophan**.

An adequate supply of dietary protein is of utmost importance in order to maintain optimal health, growth, function and rejuvenation of the body. Symptoms of protein deficiency are many and varied, ranging from hair loss, brittle nails and rough skin to fatigue, anaemia and low sex drive. In addition to creating protein, various amino acids, both essential and non-essential, have been found to have specific beneficial effects on health, and these amino acids are available as nutritional supplements.

PSYLLIUM, PLANTAIN
(*PLANTAGO OVATA, PLANTAGO MAJOR*)

Psyllium is a perennial herb which is mainly cultivated in Asia. The seeds are rich in both mucilaginous substances and **fibre**. The leaves of *P. major*, the greater or common plantain, which grows prolifically as a weed throughout the British Isles, also contain tannins. Psyllium is an intestinal lubricant that soothes the digestive tract and is beneficial in cases of internal infections, ulcers and diverticulosis. It is also an astringent and its decoctions, which promote blood-clotting, are used on wounds and haemorrhoids. However, its most common use is in fighting constipation. Mixed with water, the powdered seeds make an excellent laxative as, like **bran**, they absorb water in the intestine and swell, stimulating a natural bowel movement. Psyllium husk powder in bulk and capsule form is available in health food shops.

PULSES SEE LEGUMES

PUMPKIN (*Cucurbita*)

Pumpkin is a sweet vegetable which probably originated in North America, where it is still widely grown and eaten. It provides a good source of **beta carotene, calcium, iron** and some **B vitamins** and can also help to regulate **blood sugar** levels, and is thus of benefit to hypoglycaemics. Pumpkin promotes the expulsion of mucus from the throat, bronchi and lungs, and its regular use is said to benefit bronchial asthma. Pumpkin seeds are rich in **zinc**, and are known for their ability to destroy parasitic intestinal worms, in both children and adults.

PYCNOGENOL

Pycnogenol is the trade name for a group of **bioflavonoids** called proanthocyanidins. Although these flavonoids can be extracted from various foods such as fruits, **grains**, vegetables and grape seeds, pycnogenol is derived under patent, from the French maritime pine tree (*Pinus maritima*).

The proanthocyanidins in pycnogenol are powerful **antioxidants** and free radical scavengers. In this respect, pycnogenol is a supernutrient supplement. It has been found to be 50 times better than **vitamin E** and 20 times better than **vitamin C** in scavenging free radicals. Pycnogenol has anti–ageing properties and is usually taken to boost the immune response and prevent the degenerative diseases of ageing, such as cancer, atherosclerosis, heart attack, arthritis and diabetes.

PYRIDOXINE SEE VITAMIN B6

PYRUVATE

A new dietary supplement in health food stores, pyruvate is a salt of pyruvic acid, a naturally occuring carbohydrate found in the body and diet. Abundant in foods such as red **apples, beer**, red **wines** and certain cheeses, it is formed in the body as a by-product of carbohydrate metabolism, during the breakdown of **glucose** to ATP – the energy compound stored mostly in muscles.

Pyruvate has been researched for 25 years, and although it was initially known among athletes and bodybuilders to increase **exercise** endurance, promote fat loss and regulate **blood sugar**, over 100 health benefits were claimed for it. These include enhancement of weight loss and prevention of weight gain with overeating; protecting the heart and increasing its efficiency; reducing blood sugar level in diabetics; lowering **cholesterol**; inhibiting cancer growth and scavenging free radicals. Several studies showed that in strenuous training before competitions, pyruvate dramatically extended athletic performance by increasing glucose and glycogen stores in muscles. In these studies a mixture of pyruvate and dihydroxyacetone (DHAP) was used. In daily doses of 6 g given to obese women on a 2,000 **calorie**-a-day diet, pyruvate was found to reduce fat accumulation in the liver, promoting both fat loss and weight loss, while increasing muscle mass. Other studies showed that pyruvate lowers blood **lipids**, increases heart efficiency, improves glucose metabolism in diabetics, curbs **appetite**, increases the conversion of food to energy and acts as a powerful antioxidant.

Pyruvate is available as capsules, powder or drinks, and the Recommended Daily Allowence is 2–5 g, divided into two daily doses.

QUERCETIN

A bioflavonoid, which is becoming increasingly popular, quercetin serves as a backbone for other flavonoids and is considered to be the most active of them all. Quercetin has a wide range of beneficial effects. It has been found to be a powerful **antioxidant**, neutralizes free radicals, which are the underlying causes of the degenerative diseases of ageing such as heart disease, cancer and arthritis; it has also been reported to possess strong and prolonged anti-inflammatory and wound-healing properties. In addition, it is reported to be effective against viruses, especially oral herpes.

Quercetin has also been shown to have anti-cancer properties, and studies have revealed that it can inhibit the proliferation of malignant cells in breast and ovarian cancers and leukaemia. It has also been found to inhibit histamine release, making it useful in the treatment of allergies. Additional studies have reported on the ability of quercetin to delay the onset of cataract, and, since it is able to enhance insulin secretion, it is also useful in the control of diabetes.

Quercetin is abundant in fruits and vegetables such as citrus rind, **garlic, onions** and **blue-green algae**, and supplements of quercetin are now available in health food shops in capsule form.

Caution: High doses of quercetin supplements may cause diarrhoea.

QUINOA (*Chenopodium quinoa*)

A grain, which thrives in the high, cold altitudes of the
Andes Mountains of South America where it has been
grown for thousands of years, it was one of the staple
foods of the Aztecs and was known as the 'mother grain'.

The **protein** content of quinoa is the highest of any
of the **grains**, both in quantity and in quality. 100 g of quinoa
provide 14 g protein. It also contains more fat than other
grains, and has more **calcium** than **milk**. In addition, it is
a very good source of **iron, B vitamins, vitamin E** and
phosphorus. The grain is still cultivated in the Andes, and
remains one of the chief foods
of Andean Indians. It is also exported to the USA, where
it is processed and marketed as grain, flour or pasta.

Quinoa can be cooked in the same way as other grains,
such as **rice**; it is also included in breakfast cereals.

R

RADISH (*Raphanus sativus*)

An annual plant, cultivated for its succulent tubers, radish is eaten raw and mainly used in salads. It is an astringent and diuretic, and is used to promote **bile** flow.

Radishes and their juice are an old home remedy for coughs, rheumatism and gall bladder problems. The leaves of the plant, which are usually discarded, are very nutritious, containing almost 10 times as much **vitamin C** as the roots. They are also rich in **calcium, iron, sodium, phosphorus, sulphur** and **potassium**. In Yemenite folk medicine, radishes are used to eliminate kidney stones. Half a cup of fresh radish juice each morning on an empty stomach usually dissolves even the most stubborn stones, passing them out of the body in the urine.

Caution: Large kidney stones can scratch the urinary passage and cause bleeding as they are passed out. Two tablespoons of **olive oil** can supply lubrication and ease the elimination. Radishes are not recommended for people with gastro-intestinal inflammations or ulcers.

RASPBERRY (*Rubus idaeus*)

A widespread shrubby plant which grows wild, raspberry is cultivated for its red berries. It is an effective astringent and the leaves are rich in **vitamins, minerals** and fragarine, a substance which prevents uterine contractions.

Infusion of the leaves can be used to prevent premature labour and painful menstruation. Fresh raspberry juice is an excellent cooling beverage for fevers.

Raspberry leaf **tea**, which is available from health food stores as tea bags, can be used to stop diarrhoea, treat stomach and intestinal ulcers, and help with the healing of wounds. It is also used as a gargle.

RAW JUICE FASTING SEE FASTING

RDA (*RECOMMENDED DAILY ALLOWANCES*)

These are the amounts of **vitamins** and **minerals** required on a daily basis by the average adult. The RDA values have been created by calculating the amounts of nutrients in average diets and then adding a 'margin of safety'. However, RDA values tend to be set extremely low and have been challenged by many nutritional authorities, especially as RDAs represent average amounts for populations, rather than individuals, and people are biochemically very different from each other. For example, some people burn vitamins quicker than others, and some may have absorption defects of certain nutrients and therefore need an additional intake of these nutrients.

Initially, RDAs were intended to prevent nutrient deficiencies, but today the major public trend is towards optimal nutrition, which provides an optimal feeling of well-being and an optimal lifespan. This is the reason why many people use nutritional supplements, sometimes supplementing their diets many times above the RDA levels.

REISHI (*GANODERMA LUCIDUM*)

This is an exceptional Chinese **mushroom** that has long been highly rated in traditional Chinese medicine as a cure-all and has been used in the treatment of a variety of disorders. It is believed to promote health and longevity and to be the best booster of the body's immunity against diseases. Reishi contains **germanium** and is considered to have a powerful effect against tumours and cancers. Recent research has found reishi to be beneficial in relieving fatigue and stress, treating viral infections and joint inflammations, lowering high **cholesterol** and triglycerides, reducing heart disease symptoms, regenerating the liver, alleviating allergies, calming the nervous system, helping with the treatment of diabetes and reducing the side effects of chemotherapy.

Reishi mushrooms (available from health food stores as capsules) are now increasingly incorporated as an ingredient in many multivitamin–mineral supplements.

RENNIN, CHYMOSIN

Rennin, or chymosin, is a protein-splitting enzyme which is used to coagulate **milk** in the making of cheese. It is contained in rennet, a substance found in the lining of calves' stomachs. Rennin is used to make the milk separate into curds and **whey**. The curds are then pressed to drain off the whey and, at this point, they can form a soft cheese, such as cottage cheese, or be allowed to mature to form the harder cheeses.

RETINOL

Retinol is the fat-soluble, absorbable form of **vitamin A** which is present only in animal food (especially liver), **fish**, dairy foods and **eggs**. It is thought to serve as a precursor to two active forms of vitamin A, retinal and retinoic acid. Retinal is mainly involved with improving vision and reproduction, while retinoic acid performs the other duties of vitamin A, such as proper growth and skin health. Ninety per cent of the body's retinol is stored in the liver.

The vegetable form of vitamin A, **beta carotene** or provitamin A, cannot be used as such and must first be converted in the body to retinol.

RHODIOLA (*Rhodiola rosea*)

Native to Russia and Scandinavia, rhodiola root has been used for centuries to help people cope with the Siberian climate. Indeed, it was found to promote **serotonin**, the 'feel good' hormone. Pilot studies showed that it alleviates stress, reduces fatigue and aids heart function. Available from health food stores.

RHUBARB (*Rheum palmatum*)

A perennial vegetable that grows wild in China, it is used mainly for its roots and rhizomes. As an **appetite** stimulant and astringent, rhubarb is effective for both constipation and diarrhoea, depending on the amounts used. Large amounts can promote diarrhoea while tiny amounts will have a constipative effect.

Caution: The leaves are high in **oxalic acid**, which can bind with **calcium** and promote calcium crystals in people susceptible to kidney stones.

RICE (*ORYZA*)

Rice is a cereal grain, which is one of the world's most important food crops. It forms the main diet of more than half of the world's population, most of whom live in Asia, from where the grain is thought to have originated. It thrives in the warm, wet climates of tropical areas and is available in several types and shapes. Natural rice is a rich source of the **B vitamins, vitamin E, fibre** and unsaturated fatty acids, but unfortunately refining removes most of these nutrients – wholegrain brown rice is both nutritious and easily digestible, while white rice is nutritionally inferior.

Rice is the least allergenic of the cereal **grains** and is well tolerated even by infants and people with digestive disorders. It provides a good home remedy for diarrhoea, nausea and diabetes. Its B vitamins nourish the nervous system and help to relieve depression; it is also used by coeliacs because it does not contain **gluten**.

Short grain rice has a nuttier flavour and a thicker consistency and is better for nervousness than the long-grain, which is less sticky. Basmati rice is slightly aromatic and lighter in texture than other varieties, making it more suitable for the overweight. Wild rice, which is known to benefit the kidneys and bladder, is a grass native to North America and is more related to **corn** than to rice.

Rice can also be sprouted and used for people with weak digestion and poor **appetite**. (See SPROUTS.)

ROSE HIPS (*ROSA CANINA*)

Shiny red oval berries, rose hips are the fruits of the dog rose
and grow wild in hedgerows all over Europe and America
between August and November. Exceedingly rich in **vitamin
C**, one cup of 30 berries contains as much vitamin C as 40
oranges! Rose hips also contain **vitamins A, D** and **E** and
have a powerful antioxidant activity. Rose hip infusions have
been traditionally used for various conditions such as colds,
headaches, dizziness and mouth sores. They are mild laxatives
and useful as nerve tonics; new studies have also shown that
powdered rose hips can help reduce the pain of osteoarthritis
better than paracetamol. Dried rose hips are available in
tea bags for infusions or as a dried powder in vitamin C
supplements. **Caution:** The seeds of fresh rose hips can
irritate the mouth and stomach and should be discarded.

ROSEMARY (*ROSMARINUS OFFICINALIS*)

A beautiful, fragrant evergreen shrub which is native to the
Mediterranean regions, it has a variety of herbal uses. An
infusion of the leaves and flowering tops is a sedative that
can be used to relieve flatulence and headaches, promote
perspiration, increase **bile** flow and stimulate menstruation.
Rosemary, especially its young leaves, contains carnosic acid, a
powerful antioxidant. Recent research identified rosemary as
one of the first plants that can improve memory by inhibiting
acetylcholinesterase (a brain chemical which switches off
the connection between nerve cells). Rosemary leaves are
used as a culinary seasoning and to make essential oils for
aromatherapy. They are also used externally, mainly in
shampoos and other hair preparations.

ROYAL JELLY

A bee product, royal jelly is a thick, milky substance that is produced by young nurse bees from pollen and **honey**. It is the food that converts a regular 'worker' bee to a 'queen' bee, who is then able to lay **eggs** and reproduce. Royal jelly contains the **B vitamins**, and is particularly rich in **pantothenic acid**, the **B vitamin** that relieves stress and promotes fertility and healthy reproduction. Royal jelly also contains **vitamins A, C, D** and **E**, together with **minerals**, hormones, a vast number of **amino acids**, and antibiotic and antibacterial components, not all of which are isolated.

Royal jelly is known to strengthen the immune system and to help in such conditions as fatigue, low sex drive, liver disease, stomach ulcers, kidney disease and skin problems. Royal jelly spoils easily, and is therefore usually sold blended with honey, or in capsules. It is best kept refrigerated and taken on an empty stomach.

RUE (*Ruta graveolens*)

An aromatic, perennial plant native to the Mediterranean countries, it is also widely cultivated elsewhere. The aromatic leaves are high in **rutin**, the bioflavonoid that strengthens capillaries and blood vessels. An infusion of the leaves is diuretic, slightly increases blood pressure and has an abortifacient effect (induces abortion). In Yemenite folk medicine, rue is used to treat nervous breakdowns and to stimulate the onset of delayed menstruation.

Caution: Rue must not be taken during pregnancy. Available from specialist ethnic grocers and herbalists.

RUTIN

Rutin is a crystalline glucoside, a **bioflavonoid** closely related to hesperidin. It is present in many plants but its richest source is **buckwheat**. Rutin strengthens fragile capillaries and blood vessels, inhibits internal haemorrhages, reduces blood pressure and increases blood circulation to the hands and feet. It is also used in the treatment of haemorrhoids. Rutin is an antioxidant and can help to prevent radiation damage: its action is greatly increased when combined with **vitamin C**. Rutin is available in capsules as a supplement.

RYE (*SECALE CEREALE*)

A cereal grain widely grown in the cool climates of northern Europe, Asia, and North America, it formed the major ingredient of the bread eaten in medieval Europe. Rye is a very nourishing hard grain, regarded by many as nutritionally superior to **wheat**. It is high in **protein, calcium** and **iron**, and is a good source of **vitamins B1, B2** and niacin. Rye bread increases strength and stamina, cleans arteries, prevents anaemia, and aids the growth of hair and nails. Rich in **fluorine**, rye **sprouts** or soaked rye flakes can strengthen teeth enamel and help bone formation. Rye flour is ideally suited to making sourdough bread. Widely available.

S

SAFFLOWER SEED AND OIL

Safflower (*Carthanus tinctorius*) is an annual grain cultivated in the USA and Europe. A **tea** made from the flowers is diuretic and increases perspiration. Of all the kitchen oils, safflower oil is highest in polyunsaturated fatty acids. Its 79 per cent polyunsaturates, which contain essential fatty acids such as Linoleic acid (LA) and Gamma Linolenic acid (GLA), are known to lower **cholesterol** levels and prevent heart attacks and strokes. However, this is only a nutritional asset when the oil is fresh because the higher its content of unsaturates, the more vulnerable an oil is to oxidation and rancidity and, once rancid, the unsaturated fatty acids are converted to irritating substances. Widely available.

SAFFRON (*CROCUS SATIVUS*)

A small perennial plant cultivated in many parts of the world, including Europe and Asia, saffron is both an expensive aromatic spice and a medical herb with several benefits. Traditionally, its flower stigmas are a well-known aphrodisiac. Saffron is also believed to strengthen the **appetite**, soothe the alimentary canal, increase **bile** flow, clear liver stagnancy, help menopausal difficulties and relieve phlegm. In small doses, saffron has been used to treat coughs, bloated stomach, colic and insomnia, and it is sometimes used in herb liqueurs as an **appetite** stimulant. Widely available.

Caution: Saffron contains a poison that can damage the kidneys and nerves, and 10 g can be a fatal dose for humans. It should therefore be used only in small amounts.

SAGE (*Salvia officinalis*)

A perennial shrub that grows wild in the Mediterranean regions, sage is also widely cultivated for its culinary and medicinal properties. Traditionally used to improve mental acuity, new research now suggests that sage may restore mental functions and improve memory. Sage **tea** is astringent, sedative and expels gas; it clears the respiratory tract, makes a good gargle for sore throats and helps overcome colds. Sage is useful for night sweats as it reduces sweating. It also reduces milk flow in nursing mothers prior to weaning, prevents the formation of kidney stones by dissolving residues of uric acid, and regularizes menstruation. An infusion of sage can be applied to the scalp to reduce dandruff. Widely available.

SALMON

The salmon is a **fish** with the least saturated fat and **cholesterol**. It contains a valuable source of the highly beneficial **omega-3 fatty acids**, EPA and DHA. These essential fatty acids are effective in preventing serious cardiovascular conditions, such as hardening of the arteries, blood clots, hypertension, high cholesterol levels, heart attacks and strokes.

SALMONELLA

Salmonella is a bacteria that can be found in spoiled foods, raw **eggs**, unpasteurized **milk**, and also in the intestines of animals. It is the commonest cause of food poisoning and is mainly contracted from contaminated foods, particularly eggs, chicken and **meat** products – poorly cooked meats are a great risk. It is also easily transmitted by unhygienic food preparation, storing and handling, and unclean cutlery or cooking utensils. The effects of salmonella poisoning can vary in severity and range from diarrhoea, cramps and vomiting to fever and infections, and these can sometimes be fatal, particularly in those whose immune system is weak, such as infants and the elderly.

SALT

The richest contributor of **sodium** in the average diet, table or culinary salt has been indiscriminately condemned as a risky food, leaving many people confused about its use. It should be remembered, however, that in the right amounts, sodium is a much-needed mineral in the body. For example, it stimulates the kidneys and also gastric juices, enabling proper digestion; it promotes sweating and energy, helps to maintain a proper acid-alkaline balance and assists the transmission of nerve messages (see SODIUM).

Salt has been incriminated for increasing water retention and elevating blood pressure. Until recently, people who were overweight or hypertensive, and those with heart conditions, were warned to avoid salt and many were put on sodium-free diets. However, a new study of thousands of hypertensive patients has shown that reducing salt intake is unnecessary, unless people are aged over 45 and suffer from high blood pressure. Lowering the salt intake of younger people, even with hypertension, has been found to be of limited value. The study recommends instead that patients should take more **exercise** and drink less alcohol. The harmful effects of severe salt restriction on a large scale are only now becoming appreciated.

SAMe (S-ADENOSYLMETHIONINE)

SAMe is naturally formed in the body by reacting **methionine** and ATP (the energy molecule). SAMe acts as a principal methyl donor in the body (with **folic acid** and **vitamin B12**), donating methyl molecules (CH3) necessary to keep in check toxic levels of **homocysteine**. Since this process called methylation occurs in every cell of the body, insufficient CH3 can disrupt many biological functions. It can damage DNA and lead to increased cancer risk. It adversely affects many vital processes such as energy production, brain chemistry, heart function and liver health. Increased methylation with supplements of SAMe (400–1,000 mg/day) have been shown by various studies to support cartilage, benefit people with osteoarthritis, and provide substantial pain relief.

SARSAPARILLA (*SMILAX OFFICINALIS*)

A tropical perennial plant, which is found wild in South America, its root is used to make root **beer**, a popular beverage in North America, particularly in the American Midwest. A **tea** prepared from the root has both tonic and diuretic properties, and is used to expel gas and increase perspiration. It is also said to help in the treatment of colds, fevers, gout and rheumatism. In Spanish folk medicine, sarsaparilla was claimed to have a regenerative effect on the genital organs, and was used to help the treatment of venereal diseases such as syphilis and gonorrhoea. Available from health food stores, herbalists and as formulas.

SASSAFRAS (*SASSAFRAS ALBIDUM*)

A tree of the **laurel** family, it grows wild in the eastern
and Pacific north-west regions of the USA. A **tea** prepared

from the bark is a strong stimulant and was used by the
American Indians as an aphrodisiac. An infusion promotes
perspiration and urination, purifies the blood, and is used
in conditions such as gout, rheumatism and arthritis.

Sassafras **tea** was once popular as a tonic drink. Available
from larger health food stores and herbalists.

SAUERKRAUT

A healthy **probiotic** food, sauerkraut is made by
fermenting (pickling) **cabbage**, with or without **salt**. It is
easily made at home by crushing raw cabbage and storing
it in a ceramic or glass container for about a week.
Cabbage can be combined with a variety of herbs and
vegetables, such as **garlic, carrots** or **seaweeds**, to produce
different types of sauerkraut, which can be stored in the
refrigerator for several months, although the salted variety
has a longer storage life.

Sauerkraut can regenerate the intestines and rejuvenate
the body by increasing the intestinal flora; it balances stomach
secretions and improves digestion. Saltless sauerkraut helps
to maintain a correct acid–alkali balance, strengthen the
immune system, improve resistance to disease, stimulate blood
formation, and increase energy and well-being. For best
results, sauerkraut should be eaten on a daily basis by adding a
small amount to meals.

SAW PALMETTO (*SERENOA SERRULATA*)

A small palm tree that grows wild in coastal regions of
North America, it is also known as 'dwarf palm'. Saw
palmetto was traditionally used as a food by the south-

eastern American Indians, and it has recently made headlines in
the media as a treatment for enlarged prostate in men.

The therapeutic value of saw palmetto lies in its berries,
which contain an unusual mix of fatty acids, phytosterols and
alcohols, that have been found to have a beneficial effect on
the size and health of the prostate. This is a muscular gland
that surrounds the urethra of males at the base of the bladder,
and it becomes enlarged when its cells reproduce quicker
than normal as a result of over-secretion of hormones. This
can be due to age-related changes, so that enlargement of the
prostate gland can be a potential problem for any man over 50.
Enlargement of the prostate can produce several uncomfortable
symptoms such as difficult or frequent urination, interrupted
sleep patterns due to frequent night-time visits to the
bathroom, or incomplete emptying of the bladder. In extreme
cases, the prostate can develop inflammation or cancer.

Saw palmetto berries have been found to inhibit the
hormonal secretion of the prostate and relieve much of the
discomfort. Saw palmetto extracts are available in capsule
form at health food shops. The normal recommended dose is
160 mg, taken once or twice daily.

SEAWEEDS

Seaweeds, or marine algae, is a general descriptive name for
sea vegetables. They are extremely rich in **iodine** and in

other **minerals**, such as **calcium, iron**, and **fluorine**, and have been known for centuries for their ability to promote health. They are especially beneficial to thyroid function, and can also lower **cholesterol**, alkalize the blood, remove radioactivity residues, help with weight loss and are important in bone mineralization and density. Seaweeds are

used to treat conditions such as goitre, water retention (oedema) and swollen lymph glands. They come in several colours – brown, red, green, blue-green and yellow-green – each of which has its own individual properties in addition to the properties common to all. The most commonly used seaweeds include **kelp, agar, dulse**, hijiki, **kombu**, arame, **wakame, nori** and **Irish moss**.

SELENIUM

Selenium is a trace element that works best when combined with **vitamin E**. It is needed by the body to form **glutathione** peroxidase, an important **antioxidant** enzyme that protects the body from the damaging effects of free radicals and prevents the degenerative diseases of ageing. In fact, selenium deficiency is a known factor in premature ageing, heart attacks and cancer, and it has been estimated that if the majority of people took selenium supplements, the incidence of cancer could be reduced by 70 per cent! In conjunction with **vitamin E**, selenium helps the body to eliminate toxic elements such as **lead, cadmium** and **mercury**.

The beneficial effects of selenium are many and varied. It increases immunity to diseases, slows down ageing, alleviates menopausal discomfort, promotes energy and sexual potency, and helps to prevent auto-immune diseases such as arthritis and multiple sclerosis, and degenerative diseases such as cancer and atherosclerosis.

Some of the deficiency symptoms of selenium are manifested as fatigue, susceptibility to infections, premature ageing, predisposition to cancer and low sexual potency – selenium is concentrated in the male sex glands and is lost in ejaculated semen. Dietary sources of selenium are limited as plants do not require selenium for growth and can happily prosper in selenium-poor soils. Among the best natural sources are **brewer's yeast**, raw wheat germ, tuna, **onions**, nuts and seeds. An average daily consumption for adults of 50–200 mcg is recommended, with a range of 50–80 mcg for children. Selenium is available as a supplement in health food shops.

SENNA (*CASSIA ACUTIFOLIA*)

The dried pods and leaves of the cassia tree, which grows wild in North African countries, senna contains two active glycosides and is a well-known remedy for chronic constipation. An infusion of the leaves and pods will act as a strong laxative. Senna is often combined with other substances to eliminate intestinal worms; it can also help to counteract bad breath. Available from health food stores and widely incorporated in laxative formulas.

Caution: Senna should not be used in cases of haemorrhoids.

SERINE SEE PHOSPHATIDYLSERINE(PS)

SEROTONIN

Serotonin has recently been receiving considerable media attention for its many beneficial effects. It is one of the **neurotransmitters**, i.e. brain chemicals that carry messages between the nerve cells, and unlike other excitatory neurotransmitters, such as adrenalin, serotonin is an inhibiting or calming neurotransmitter and reduces brain

cell activity. It counteracts depression, anxiety and fear, lifting the spirits; it also increases libido, induces sleep, improves memory and concentration, supresses the **appetite** and aids weight reduction. In fact, drugs which raise serotonin levels are now being used to help with weight loss.

Unfortunately, serotonin cannot be taken as a supplement because it is broken down during digestion. It is derived in the body from the amino acid **tryptophan** which is abundant in foods such as **milk** and bananas. Starchy foods such as **potatoes**, pasta and breads can also help to raise serotonin levels by increasing insulin, which in turn raises tryptophan levels.

SESAME SEEDS (*Sesamum indicum*)

A annual herb that originated in Africa or India, it is now widely cultivated in the tropical regions of China, India, Japan, Mexico and the south-western states of the United States.

Sesame seeds are very nutritious and provide an excellent source of **protein, calcium**, omega-6 fatty acids, **magnesium, iron, zinc, vitamins A** and **E** and niacin. Available hulled or unhulled, the unhulled seeds – as used

in breads or grain dishes – are more nutritious because
most of the mineral content of the seed is contained in
the hull. The hull is high in minerals. However, the hull
also contains aflatoxins and oxalic acid which deplete
calcium. Hulled sesame seeds are purer, safer, more
digestible and more alkaline. Hulled sesame seeds are
commonly available as sesame butter, called tahini, which
can be used in a number of ways. Combined with **honey**,
tahini makes a delicious spread; blended with **water,
lemon** and **garlic**, it provides a base for a healthy
salad dressing which is very popular in the Middle
East. Allowed to stand for a while, the oil separates from
tahini and can be used as an excellent cooking oil; it can
also be used externally to soothe skin problems. Tahini
can be combined with water to prepare sesame milk,
which isused to lubricate the intestines, to help relieve
constipation, and is also recommended for stiff joints,
weak knees, nervous spasms and increasing milk secretion
in nursing mothers.

SHIITAKE (*LENTINULA EDODES*)

A prized mushroom used in the Chinese tradition for
its health benefits shiitake is a rich source of **selenium**
and **iron**, but its acclaimed health benefits a e due its
polysaccharide content, particularly to lentinan, an active
compound with the ability to boost immunity (by increasing
proliferation of T cells), to help fight infection and to exert
an anti-cancer activity. Shiitake is now cultivated and
widely available.

SHEPHERD'S PURSE (*CAPSELLA BURSA-PASTORIS*)

A widespread annual herb, growing wild throughout
Europe, particularly in poor soils and wastelands, it is rich
in **calcium, sodium**, and **vitamins C** and **K**. The whole
plant has medicinal properties and is an effective blood
coagulant, which can be used to stop bleeding, both
external and internal, including excessive menstrual
bleeding. It is also a diuretic. Available from health food
stores and incorporated in nutritional formulas.

SHORT-CHAIN FATTY ACIDS (SCFA)

SCFAs are produced naturally in the intestines from dietary
fibre by the intestinal flora. The three SCFAs, acetic acid,
propionic acid and butyric acid, have important functions.
Acetate and propionate are stored in the liver and used for
energy production. Butyrate is an important energy source
for the metabolic activity of the colon. It has effective
anti-cancer effects and is thought to be responsible for the
cancer-inhibiting properties of dietary fibre. Butyrate is also
used in enemas in the treatment of ulcerative colitis.

Different fibres produce differing amounts of SCFAs in
the colon. **Pectins** from **apples, guar gum** and legume
fibres produce more SCFAs than oat **bran** or **corn** fibre.

SHOYU

A **wheat**-containing type of soy sauce, shoyu is a
traditional Japanese seasoning made from **soybeans,
wheat, salt** and koji (a fermentation starter made from a
special yeast culture, aspergillus oryzae). The fermentation

of shoyu usually takes a few months. It is commonly used to salt and flavour foods.

Caution: People with an allergy to wheat or coeliacs should not use shoyu. Instead they can use **tamari**.

SILICON

Although, as a constituent of sand and rocks, silicon is the most abundant element contained in the earth's crust, in the human body it is found in only trace amounts as silica (silicon dioxide). In spite of this small overall amount, however, silica is present in almost every tissue of the body and is essential for cell growth. It is especially concentrated in the hair, nails and connective tissues such as the skin. It can inhibit the greying of hair, keep the skin smooth and supple and prevent brittle nails. For these reasons, it is incorporated into many cosmetic formulas. However, a distinction should be made between water-soluble silica and the controversial silicone breast implants. Despite the similarity in the name, natural silica differs considerably from breast implant silicone, which is an industrial polymer containing controversial hydrocarbons suspected of being carcinogenic.

Silica and silica gel have been reported to be beneficial in treating many disorders, including heartburn, ulcers, gastritis, colitis, varicose veins, bronchitis, arteriosclerosis, gum recession, allergic rashes and many others.

The best natural sources of silica include **horsetail** herb, **oats**, millet, **barley, onions**, whole **wheat** and red **beet**. Silica supplements, for both internal and external use, are available from health food shops in many forms, such as effervescent or chewable tablets, capsules, powders and silica gel. All come with directions for use.

SLIPPERY ELM SEE ELM

SOD

This very important antioxidant enzyme, which includes **copper** and **zinc**, is found naturally within cells. It protects cells and tissues from the damage of superoxide free radicals and is a general anti-ageing enzyme. It is reported to be especially helpful in preventing the damage to joints, membranes and lubricating fluids that occurs in rheumatoid arthritis. It also helps to prevent cataracts.

SOD is available as a supplement although, when taken orally, it is mostly destroyed in the digestive tract. However, when administered by injection, it is reported to have been beneficial for both osteoarthritis and rheumatoid arthritis.

SODIUM

The main component of **salt** is sodium, a mineral prevalent in the body that is found mainly in the fluids surrounding body cells rather than within them. Sodium is highly important in maintaining osmotic pressure in tissues, enabling oxygen and nutrients to move in or out of cells; it stimulates the kidneys and keeps **calcium** soluble, preventing kidney stones; it also stimulates the secretion of gastric juices, helping digestion, promotes sweating and helps to prevent heatstroke, and improves feelings of lassitude in people with low blood pressure. Together with **potassium**, it participates in nerve transmissions and maintains a correct acid – alkaline balance.

Excessive sodium tends to elevate blood pressure, constrict

blood vessels and cause water retention, resulting in oedema and hypertension. People with high blood pressure, heart disease, oedema, or those who are over- weight, are usually advised to avoid salt and use low- sodium diets. This can be done by using potassium-based salt substitutes, as well as herb powders such as **celery, basil, caraway, mustard** or **parsley**.

Salt deficiency is very uncommon, but can occur as a result of excessive perspiration. Some of the best natural sources include table salt, **kelp** and **seaweeds, meats**, beets, **carrots**, chard and **dandelion** greens.

Caution: Excessive sodium intake should be balanced by increased potassium, since sodium causes the excretion of potassium in the urine.

SORBITOL

Sorbitol is a type of sugar, that is commercially refined from **glucose** and sucrose. It is about 60 per cent as sweet as sugar and is popular among diabetics since it does not raise insulin levels as sharply as table sugar. Most sorbitol is converted in the body to carbon dioxide and **fructose**, with only a small part of it being converted to glucose; this is then absorbed through the intestines over a relatively long period of time so that a sharp insulin release is not triggered as is the case with table sugar. Since insulin is known to promote detrimental changes in the cardiovascular system, sorbitol is therefore a much more desirable sweetener than ordinary sugar, even for healthy people. In addition, the slow metabolism of sorbitol does not tax the sugar-balancing glands and causes much less tooth decay. Sorbitol also increases the absorption of certain **vitamins**, such as B12, which is why it is included in many multi-vitamin tablets.

SOYBEAN

An ancient staple crop of Asia, the soybean is a legume noted for its high vegetable **protein** content (38 per cent), which is greater than the protein content of **milk**. The crop has long been considered a solution to famine in Asia, since an acre of soybeans produces 20 times more usable protein than the same acreage used for grazing beef or growing fodder.

In recent years, soybeans have developed into one of the world's major sources of vegetable oil and texturized vegetable protein (TVP) and, as such, they are included in many foods, including ice cream, soy sauce, beansprouts and **tofu**. Soya milk does not contain the saturated fat, **cholesterol** and toxic residues of dairy milk. It has, to a large extent, replaced dairy milk in many people's diets and revolutionized their eating habits.

Soybeans have been found to be a storehouse of phytochemicals – beneficial antioxidant nutrients, such as saponins, phytosterols and phenolic acids – which protect the body from free radical damage, reducing the risk of the degenerative diseases of ageing, such as heart attack, cancer and strokes. Two of the best anticarcinogens in soya are some plant oestrogens, which prevent breast cancer, and **genistein**, which inhibits the growth of cancer cells. In fact, soybeans have a mild oestrogenic activity due to their **isoflavones**, also called phytoestrogens. Eating soya products can therefore be beneficial for women in HRT and can help offset some postmenopausal symptoms. Soy beans have also been found to be beneficial in reducing cholesterol levels and preventing heart attack. A new Canadian University study found that three glasses of soya milk and one soya dessert consumed daily lowered the 'bad' **LDL cholesterol** by 11 per cent and increased the 'good' **HDL** by 9 per cent in 70 per cent of the subjects. Research has shown that the substitution of soya products in the daily diet for just part of the normal **meat** and dairy milk intake can provide a number of health benefits. All widely available. (See also SPROUTS.)

SPINACH (*Spinacia oleracea*)

A popular garden vegetables native to south-east Asia, spinach is an excellent source of **iron, calcium**, chlorophyll, **beta carotene** (provitamin A), **vitamin C**, riboflavin, **sodium** and **potassium**. It is a diuretic and laxative, and can also be used to stop minor haemorrhaging such as nosebleeds. As it is rich in **iron** and chlorophyll, spinach builds the blood, while its **sulphur** content helps to clean the liver and relieve herpes irritations. In addition, its **vitamin A** content can help to prevent night blindness. Although spinach provides an exceptional source of calcium, it is also high in **oxalic acid**, which can partly interfere with the absorption of the calcium.

Caution: People with a tendency to kidney stones should eat spinach sparingly since its high oxalic acid can tend to form calcium-oxalate kidney stones in susceptible individuals.

SPIRULINA

Spirulina is a blue-green, single-cell algae, which is spiral-shaped – hence its name. It thrives in warm alkaline lakes such as Lake Chad in Africa and Lake Texcoco in Mexico. The algae, which appears to be a floating green scum, is collected from the lake and dried. Spirulina was so highly valued as a sustaining food by the ancient Aztecs that it was used by them as currency – and modern science has recently discovered why. Spirulina contains over 65 per cent complete **protein**, a rarity among plant foods, and this protein, which is predigested by the algae, is so well-balanced that it is easier to digest than **meat**. Spirulina absorbs and retains many **minerals**

from the lake, including **potassium, calcium, zinc, magnesium, manganese, selenium, iron** and **phosphorus**. In addition, it is a rich source of the **B vitamins**, including usable amounts of **B12**, as well as **vitamin E, beta carotene**, GLA (essential fatty acid) and chlorophyll.

Spirulina has toning and cleansing properties and can be used to detoxify the liver and kidneys, cleanse the arteries, build and enrich the blood and promote intestinal flora. It is also very beneficial for weight control, not only because it is a low-calorie nutrient, but also because it contains high amounts of **phenylalanine**, the amino acid which curbs the **appetite**.

Spirulina has been used in the treatment of anaemia, weakness, malnutrition, hepatitis, inner inflammations, diabetes, hypoglycaemia and poor skin tone. It is a versatile food supplement which strengthens the immune system and increases resistance to disease and inflammations. It also contains a blue pigment, phycocyanin, which is a protein known to inhibit cancer. Since it is grown and harvested in unpolluted areas, totally free of environmental pollutants, spirulina is one of the safest foods available. It is sold in health food shops in both powder and tablet form.

SPROUTS

Sprouts (young shoots from recently germinated seeds), mainly **soybean**, have been a part of the Chinese diet for thousands of years. Sprouts are rich in chlorophyll, **vitamins A, C, D, E, K** and **B complex**, and in **minerals** such as **calcium, phosphorus, potassium, magnesium** and **iron**. They are also abundant in quality **protein** and **enzymes**, making them easily digestible.

Sprouts have been described as 'the most living food in the world' since, unlike most plants, they are eaten at the peak of their freshness and vitality while they are still growing, and anyone who eats sprouts regularly will experience this vitality and increased energy. Sprouts are diuretics and appetizers and detoxify the body. They are used for weight loss, arthritis, oedema, peptic and duodenal ulcers, and by people with weak digestion.

Miraculous things happen when grain or legume seeds begin to germinate – the starches and oils contained in the seeds are converted to vitamins, proteins, enzymes and simple sugars. For example, vitamin C increases six-fold so that a 100 g serving of soybean sprouts will contain 120 mg vitamin C, which is double the recommended daily amount. The protein content of **alfalfa** sprouts rises to between 16 and 31 per cent, and their carotene content equals that of **carrots**. The B vitamins, enzymes and other nutrients also increase spectacularly, making sprouts an easily digested form of nourishment.

Alfalfa sprouts are among the most popular and, because they contain more minerals, they are more nutritious than other sprouts. The roots of the alfalfa plant can penetrate as deeply as 30 m (100 feet), where access to minerals is highest, and thus the sprout can contain concentrated amounts of iron, calcium, magnesium, potassium, **zinc**, phosphorus, **sodium, sulphur, silicon**, chlorine and **cobalt**.

Sprouts are commonly sold in both health food shops and supermarkets. Seeds such as **peas**, chickpeas, **wheat** sesame and **corn** are easily sprouted at home using plastic sprouters available in health food stores.

SQUASH, WINTER (*CUCURBITA*)

A gourd-shaped vegetable native to North America, winter squash provides an outstanding source of alpha and beta carotenes (provitamin A), and contains good amounts of **calcium, phosphorus** and **potassium**. Squash can benefit the stomach, reduce inflammations and improve circulation, and squash seeds are reputed to be effective in destroying worms. Some healers recommend that a handful of seeds should be eaten daily for three weeks in order to eliminate parasitic worms.

STEVIA (*STEVIA REBAUDIANA*)

Increasingly sought-after for its sweet leaves and flower buds, stevia is a small plant that grows in south-western USA and throughout Latin America, where it is called yerba dulce. Thirty times sweeter than sugar and with negligible **calories**, stevia was adopted by the Japanese, who use it widely in many processed foods.

As a herb, stevia has its own beneficial properties. One of the greatest is that unlike sugar stevia does not promote tooth decay. A study done by Hiroshima University's School of Dentistry revealed that stevia suppresses the growth of dental bacteria, in contrast to sugar which promotes dental bacteria. Other studies have shown that stevia does not interfere much with **blood sugar** regulation, and is therefore well-tolerated by both hypoglycaemics and diabetics. American studies found stevia to be a tonic and diuretic, to treat mental and physical tiredness, regulate digestion and blood pressure, and help weight loss.

Stevia is increasingly available in health food stores (especially in the USA) as a powder or liquid extract. Stevia has great sweetening power: 1–3 drops of the extract can sweeten one cup of a drink. Stevia can be used for hot drinks, cooking and baking; its sweetness is not affected by heat. Stevia is recommended as a sweetener particularly for overweight people, and for those suffering from candida (thrush) or water retention (oedema).

ST JOHN'S WORT (*HYPERICUM PERFORATUM*)

A yellow-flowered herb, which is both cultivated and found wild in the UK and Europe. One explanation for its name is that its flowers are most abundant around 24 June, the birthday of John the Baptist. Traditionally used in folk medicine, infusions of the flowers can have a beneficial effect on metabolism and **bile** secretion and can positively affect mood; they can stimulate **appetite**, improve circulation and have a general anti-inflammatory effect. A **tea** of the leaves is said to stimulate expulsion of phlegm or mucous, and is beneficial in coughs. Recent studies indicated however, that St John's wort extracts can ease the symptoms of anxiety and depression, alleviate stress,

promote sleep, boost energy and relieve PMS symptoms.
A recent pilot study showed that the herb's extract (in
daily doses of 135–235 mg) can reduce fatigue or
depression linked to tiredness. These extracts contain
0.2 per cent of the active ingredient hypericin, and capsules
made of the standardized extracts can be a natural alternative
to prescription anti depressant drugs such as Prozac, MAO
inhibitors and tricyclics. The capsules, extracts and herbs
are widely available from health food stores. Positive
benefits may be experienced within 4–6 weeks of
initial use.

STRAWBERRIES (*Fragraria*)

A delicious acidic fruit that combines well with a **protein**
meal, strawberries are an exceptional source of **vitamin C**. A
100 g serving of fresh, ripe strawberries provides 60 mg vitamin
C, more than the UK RDA. They are low in **sodium** and high
in **potassium**, a boon for hypertensive people on low-sodium
diets. They are rich in **silicon** which is useful in repairing
and strengthening connective tissue and arteries. Strawberries
are also high in **pectin**, the soluble **fibre** that helps eliminate
cholesterol. Strawberries have a strong antioxidative action
and are a useful fruit to eat in the treatment of heart and
circulatory diseases. They contain a considerable amount of an
anti-cancer compound, ellagic acid, which helps reduce the
risk of cancer. They provide modest amounts of **iron**, which
is well assimilated due to the presence of vitamin C, and they
can therefore be helpful in the treament of fatigue and anaemia.
Traditionally, strawberries were used by herbalists to treat
athritis, gout and rheumatism and to relieve urinary difficulties.
Eaten before meals, strawberries can help poor digestion. They

are best eaten fresh and ripe. If sugar needs to be sprinkled on them, then they are not ripe. Allergic reactions are often caused by eating unripe strawberries.

SUGAR SEE CARBOHYDRATES

SULPHUR

Dubbed as 'the beauty mineral', sulphur is important for smooth, glossy hair and healthy skin and nails. It is a non-metallic mineral, abundant in nature and present in every cell. It is needed for the formation of collagen, one of the most prevalent **proteins**, which is found in skin, bone and **cartilage**. As such, sulphur contributes to a healthy looking skin. It also has a laxative effect due to its ability to absorb **water** in the intestines – Epsom salts are in fact sulphates of **magnesium**.

Sulphur detoxifies the body, cleans the arteries and helps the body to rid itself of damaging toxic elements. Together with proteins, sulphur forms the vitally important sulphur-containing **amino acids cysteine, taurine** and methionine. **Cysteine** and methionine are needed to form the important anti-ageing, antioxidant **enzymes** that neutralize dangerous peroxide free radicals and help prevent the degenerative diseases of ageing, such as arthritis. In fact, sulphur has long been known to benefit arthritis, and one of its best sources is **eggs**, which are high in sulphur-containing cysteine. Used externally, in ointments and in the spa waters of regions such as the Dead Sea, sulphur has traditionally been considered beneficial for the treatment of psoriasis, eczema and dermatitis.

Deficiency symptoms of sulphur can include arthritis,

dry hair, brittle nails and rough skin. Some of the best
natural sources of the mineral are eggs, **meat, onions,
alfalfa, broccoli, cabbage** and **watercress**. (See also
MSM.)

SUNFLOWER SEED AND SUNFLOWER OIL

Sunflowers (*Helianthus*), which originated in North
America and were cultivated by the American Indians,
were first introduced into Europe in the sixteenth century.
Nowadays, vast fields of the flowers are a familiar sight across
many European landscapes in the summer months.

Sunflower seeds are sun-energized nutritional power-
houses and it is no wonder that in pre-revolutionary Russia
field soldiers received a kilo of sunflower seeds as emergency
rations on which to subsist if stranded. The seeds are rich in
protein (24 per cent), polyunsaturated fatty acids (66 per
cent), **vitamins A, E, D** and several **B vitamins, calcium,
magnesium, phosphorus, iron, zinc, potassium,
fluorine** and **iodine**.

Sunflower seeds can be used as a snack, a topping for
salads, as a nut butter spread, or can be included in bread.
The seeds have been described as beneficial to eyesight, skin
and fingernails, and are a useful adjunct in the treatment of
hypertension and irritated nerves. Sprouted sunflower seeds
are easily digestible and rich in **vitamin E, lecithin** and
pectin. As a supplement, 2 tablespoons of sunflower seeds
a day are recommended, even for people on reducing diets.
Both are widely available.

Sunflower seed oil is one of the richest sources of
essential fatty acids. It contains as much as 66 per cent
essential omega-6 fatty acids, and has the highest content of

all seeds of the essential linoleic acid. The oil can be used as an all-purpose kitchen oil, although it is best used fresh and raw as a base in salad dressings to obtain its full nutritional value. It can also be blended with **butter**, thereby enriching the butter with its essential fatty acids.

SWEET POTATOES AND YAMS (*DIOSCOREA*)

A vegetable with large, fleshy, edible roots, sweet potatoes are believed to have originated in South America. Today, they are grown throughout the world and are an important food in many countries – about 85 per cent of the world's sweet potato crop is grown in China.

Outstandingly rich in **vitamin A** (many times more so than potatoes), sweet potatoes also provide **vitamin C, calcium, iron, potassium, phosphorus** and **sodium**, but they must be baked or boiled in their skins to retain these nutrients. Due to their exceptional vitamin A content, sweet potatoes can be used to improve night vision. They are also reported to increase milk secretion in nursing mothers, remove toxins from the body and treat underweight and diarrhoea.

Sweet potatoes are best selected when fresh looking, firm to the touch, and preferably either with a dark grey skin colour (**yams**) or red skin colour (sweet potatoes) – most 'yams' sold in the USA are in fact sweet potatoes with red flesh. The vegetables should not be refrigerated as this can cause chilling injuries. However, if stored in a cool, dry place they can be kept for several months. They are widely available.

Caution: Since sweet potatoes can cause indigestion and abdominal swelling, they should be eaten in moderate servings.

T

TAHINI SEE SESAME

TAMARI

A **wheat**-free soy sauce, made from **soybeans**, sea **salt** and koji (a fermentation starter made of a special yeast culture, aspergillus oryzae), tamari is traditionally a by-product of **miso** production. It is made from the liquid that exudes from the soybean paste as the miso ferments.

Good tamari is allowed the to ferment and age for at least a year. Although similar in appearance and flavour to **shoyu**, tamari has a stronger, sharper taste and aroma. It is used instead of salt and to add complex flavour.

TAMARIND (*TAMARINDUS INDICA*)

An evergreen tree native to India, it bears small, sweet fruits in pods. Tamarind fruit is well known as a gentle laxative and is sometimes used as an ingredient in laxative preparations. The leaves are reputed to destroy parasitic intestinal worms. In Asia, tamarind fruit is eaten as a food; it is also made into a refreshing and cooling beverage, which is particularly suitable for people with fever. Tamarind is exported and is available in specialist shops in the west.

TAPIOCA

An edible starch obtained from the fleshy rootstock of the tropical cassava shrub, also called manioc, native to Central and South America. It has been the prime source of starch for the native Brazilians who gave it its name. Raw cassava contains toxic glycosides, which is why it has to be soaked and cooked. Tapioca is available in several forms, such as flakes or flour, and is widely used in puddings and as a thickener in soups and other liquid foods.

TARRAGON (*ARTEMISIA DRACUNCULUS*)

A green perennial shrub, its aromatic leaves are commonly used as a culinary herb. The fresh leaves and oil are used in tarragon **mustard** and tarragon vinegar, and also in the cooking of **fish** or chicken. Infusions of tarragon leaves can be used to stimulate digestive secretions and **appetite**, relieve digestive disorders, bring on delayed menstruation, and promote urination by stimulating the kidneys. Tarragon **tea**, taken at bedtime, can help to relieve insomnia.

TAURINE

Taurine is a **sulphur**-containing, non-essential amino acid. However, it is one of the most abundant **amino acids** in the body and an **antioxidant** that neutralizes free radicals. It also helps to raise **calcium** levels in the body by transporting calcium (and **sodium**) across the intestinal wall into the bloodstream. In addition, taurine is a component of **bile**, which is essential for the digestion of **fats**, the absorption of fat-soluble **vitamins** and for controlling **cholesterol** levels. Taurine is produced in the body from **cysteine** with the help of **vitamin B6**, and is concentrated in excitable tissues such as the heart, muscles and nerve tissues, but it is not commonly found in food. It is thought to have an inhibitory action on epilepsy and has been used to reduce seizures. Its inhibitory action can also help to counteract anxiety and stress, especially when combined with **histidine** and **glycine**. Taurine is available as a food supplement and beneficial levels range between 500 and 3,000 mg daily.

TEA (*CAMELLIA SINENSIS*)

The tea plant is an evergreen that is grown in many tropical and subtropical regions of the world, particularly in India and China, which together produce the bulk of the world's tea supplies. The flavours of the teas produced vary from country to country, and are dependent not only on soil type and processing methods, but also on the elevation of the plantations, with the finest tea coming from higher, cooler areas as the plant grows more slowly in cool air, adding to its flavour.

Black tea is a stimulating, refreshing and diuretic beverage provided it is not strongly steeped, only lightly infused. It is traditionally used to aid digestion, especially after a heavy meal; it also quenches thirst, relieves flatulence and counteracts diarrhoea. A popular tea variety, 'Earl Grey' consists of black tea blended with bergamot oil, which is in itself refreshing, relaxing and calming, and adds these properties in the blending to the tea.

Common tea contains stimulating and astringent substances, including **theophylline**, theine and tannins, which are known to stimulate overproduction of cellular products, such as fibrous tissue and cyst fluid. Strong tea is used medicinally to halt dysentery and treat chronic inflammations such as gastritis and enteritis. It is also used externally for certain skin conditions. Tea includes the **minerals sodium, potassium, magnesium, calcium** and **manganese**. In tea-drinking countries, a third or more of the daily consumption of manganese comes from tea.

Excessive drinking of tea has been found to contribute to constipation, nervousness, breast lumps and, in sensitive individuals, to mimic the many symptoms of irritable bowel syndrome.

Some milder types of tea, which are made from the branches of certain tea plants, are exported from Japan and marketed as 'bancha twig tea' or 'kukicha'. (See also GREEN TEA.)

TEA TREE OIL (*MELALEUCA ALTERNIFOLIA*)

Tea tree is a native of Australia where it is cultivated especially for its valuable oil, which is extracted from the leaves by steam distillation. This oil has been found to be an effective antiseptic, with strong germicidal and fungicidal actions.

For many years, the Australian aboriginals bathed in the healing waters of swampy areas in which the tea tree grew. They used the plant on their skins by crushing the leaves and spreading the pulp on affected areas. When discovered in 1700 by British explorers, tea tree was named by Captain Cook when he observed the aboriginals brewing tea from the leaves. Since then, the tea tree has been studied scientifically and found to contain 48 compounds, including terpine 4-ol, one of its most therapeutic ingredients. These compounds, not all of which have been identified, have been found to be beneficial in healing infected wounds, skin inflammations, carbuncles and pus-filled infections; as such, they were used during World War II by Australian troops.

Tea tree oil has since been found to be very beneficial in the treatment of various conditions such as bladder inflammation (cystitis), athlete's foot, nappy rash, insect bites, sunburn, cuts, fungi, dandruff and itchy scalp.

Nowadays, tea tree oil is incorporated into many personal care products, such as dandruff shampoos and conditioners, deodorants, toothpastes, antiseptic mouthwashes, ointments for treating acne and fungal infections, and as a douche for vaginal yeast infections.

TEMPEH

The most popular soya food in Indonesia, tempeh originated in Java more than 200 years ago and is now sold in thousands of shops in Java alone, and in increasing numbers of health food shops in the USA and other western countries.

Tempeh is a fermented soya product made from cooked **soybeans** bound together by a dense fungus (rhizopus) and then moulded into compact patties. Sold fresh, refrigerated or frozen, the patties can be sliced and fried until crisp, and their flavour and texture resemble southern-fried chicken. Different varieties of tempeh are produced by combining the soybeans with **grains** such as **wheat, rice**, millet or **coconut**.

Soya tempeh is highly nutritious. It contains 18 per cent **protein** and is an exceptional **vegetarian** source of **vitamin B12**. Popular western recipes include tempeh burgers, seasoned crisp tempeh and tempeh sandwiches.

THEOBROMINE

An ingredient found mainly in cocoa and **chocolate**, theobromine is a stimulating alkaloid and one of the methylxanthines, a group of compounds that includes **caffeine** and **theophylline**. Theobromine expands blood vessels in the heart, increases urination, reduces **calcium** absorption, and is a mild stimulator of the nervous system. It is known to stimulate overproduction of cellular products, such as fibrous tissue and cyst fluid.

THEOPHYLLINE

An alkaloid found in **tea**, theophylline is a methylxanthine, diuretic and a mild stimulator.

THIAMINE SEE VITAMIN BI

THREONINE

An essential amino acid which helps to maintain **protein** balance in the body, it is important for the synthesis of collagen. Threonine is concentrated in the heart, nervous system and skeletal muscles, and also helps the liver to handle fats in combination with **aspartic acid** and **methionine**.

THYME (*THYMUS VULGARIS*)

A small, scented garden plant native to the Mediterranean regions, thyme was used by the Romans as both a culinary and a therapeutic herb. Its aromatic and spicy tasting leaves, which are rich in essential oils, are used in cooking and in infusions. Thyme is a good tonic for the stomach and nerves. Its tea relieves flatulence, promotes **appetite**, strengthens digestion, loosens phlegm and increases perspiration. Infusions have a calming effect, relax muscle spasms and alleviate exhaustion. Extracts and infusions are also used to treat bronchitis, laryngitis and coughs. Thyme vinegar was used for centuries to relieve headaches.

Essential oil of thyme makes a good antiseptic mouthwash, and is also used externally for warts and for a relaxing bath.

Caution: Too much thyme can overstimulate the thyroid and cause poisoning symptoms.

TOCOPHEROL see VITAMIN E

TOCOTRIENOLS

This is a group of natural compounds related to tocopherols (**vitamin E**). Whereas the tocopherol molecule consists of a ring and a long saturated side chain, the tocotrienol differs by having three double-bond as their side chain. However, the tocotrienols are less widely distributed in nature. While tocopherols are found mainly in wheat germ, corn and **soybean** oils, tocotrienols are particularly rich in palm, **rice bran** and **barley** oils. Once thought to be of a lesser nutritional value, tocotrienols were found be stronger **antioxidants** than tocopherols, and to have a better effect as anti- tumour and cholesterol-reducing agents. The tocotrienols are considered to have a better penetration of fatty tissues such as brain and liver, which accounts for their improved performance.

The tocotrienols consist of alpha, beta, gamma and delta. Gamma, delta and alpha being the most used. A mix of alpha tocopherol and tocotrienols is now considered the best approach, and the first formulas are available in health food shops in capsule form.

TOFU

A common staple of Japanese cuisine, tofu is a cheese-like **soybean** curd which has now become extremely popular in western countries and various types, such as silken tofu, firm tofu or tofu puddings, are currently available in health food shops.

Tofu has been praised for its high **protein** content of 35 per cent, and for its high protein quality, which includes all the essential **amino acids**. Indeed, many people in Asia depend on tofu for their daily protein, and it is now considered a good replacement for **meat**, thus allowing more people to become **vegetarians**. As a serving of 250 g provides only 147 **calories**, it is ideal as a diet food – an equal amount of beef would contain five times the calories. Tofu is also low in saturated **fats** and **cholesterol**, but is rich in **calcium** and it is a good source of the **B vitamins, vitamin E, potassium** and **sodium**. As such, it is beneficial for conditions such as diabetes, heart disease and atherosclerosis.

Fresh tofu will keep for about five to seven days when

refrigerated; deep-fried tofu will keep up to 10 days; and special types of silken tofu can be kept sealed in their containers for up to six months. Available from health food stores and supermarkets.

TOMATOES (*LYCOPERSICON ESCULENTUM*)

Tomatoes originated in South America and were brought to Europe from Mexico in the mid-sixteenth century. Tomatoes belong to the solanum family and, historically, early varieties were high in solanine and considered poisonous until safer types were developed. They are rich in **vitamins A** and **C** and a good source of **calcium, phosphorus, potassium** and **sodium**. They detoxify the body, purify the blood, strengthen digestion and are useful in cases of poor **appetite**, poor digestion and constipation. Although tomatoes are considered an acidic food, they alkalize the blood after digestion and are useful in treating acidic conditions such as gout. Tomatoes contain **lycopene**, a powerful antioxidant carotenoid that neutralizes damaging free radicals. Lycopene has been found to be outstandingly effective in quenching singlet oxygen, which is a very reactive type of free radical that damages the **DNA** blueprint (which supervises cell division), causing mutations and cancer. In fact, the results of one study have indicated that increasing dietary lycopene levels may provide a significant protection from digestive tract cancers. Lycopene is now being incorporated as an ingredient in various multivitamin preparations.

Caution: Tomatoes can interfere with calcium absorption and should be avoided in cases of arthritis. More than four tomatoes a day are not recommended.

TRYPSIN

A protein-splitting enzyme secreted by the pancreas, trypsin enables the digestion of **proteins** in the intestines. It is included in many digestive-aid tablets such as **pancreatin**.

TRYPTOPHAN

An an essential **amino acid**, tryptophan has several crucial roles. Used in the body as a building block of **protein**, tryptophan helps manufacture antibodies, produce niacin (**vitamin B3**), and create **serotonin**, which is an inhibitory neurotransmitter – a brain chemical that conveys calming messages between brain cells. Serotonin induces sleep at night and relaxation during the day. It helps alleviate stress, reduce depression, treat insomnia, control hyperactivity in children, stabilize blood pressure and protect the heart. Moreover, an Italian study found that tryptophan (the 5-HTP form) is also useful for dieting. It can help overweight people lose weight by naturally reducing the **appetite** and carbohydrate intake, seemingly due to the release of the calming serotonin. Tryptophan needs **vitamin B6** and **C** to be converted to serotonin, and an adequate level of vitamin B3 is also important. When these are in short supply, less serotonin is available, and this can be manifested by symptoms such as insomnia, depression, anxiety and hypertension. Tryptophan rich foods include milk and bananas.

The form of tryptophan currently available from health food stores is 5-Hydroxy Tryptophan (5-HTP), derived from the beans of an African bush, *Griffonia simplicifolia*. The Recommended Daily Allowance is 100–200 mg taken between meals. (See **Genetically Modified Foods**.)

TURMERIC (*Curcuma longa*)

A common culinary spice, its source is the roots of a plant which is native to Asia. Turmeric was traditionally used by both Indian and Chinese systems of medicine to treat inflammations and cure sprains. It contains a yellow pigment, curcumin, an active ingredient that has been used for centuries not only to season foods but also as a food preservative and colouring agent. The curcuminoids in turmeric are a group of phenolic acids that have been found to have unique antioxidant and anti-inflammatory properties. They retard age-related diseases by preventing free radical damage, inhibit the growth of cancer cells, protect the liver from toxins, help to dissolve gallstones, lower **cholesterol** levels, alleviate joint swellings, increase joint flexibility and reduce menstrual pain. Studies with HIV patients have shown that turmeric also has a beneficial effect in the treatment of AIDS.

Used externally in a poultice, turmeric mixed with lime is an ancient household remedy for sprains, muscular pain and inflamed joints. It is available as a nutritional supplement in capsule form.

TURNIPS (*Brassica campestris*)

Turnips are a member of the cruciferous vegetable family, which also includes **broccoli** and **cabbage**. Although popularly considered as a starchy root vegetable, both the turnip root and its green leaves are edible. The root is rich in **vitamins A, B and C**, and **minerals** such as **sulphur, calcium, potassium, sodium** and **phosphorus**. It is also rich in **fibre** and contains far fewer calories than **potato**. A serving of 100 g has only 22 calories. Turnip greens supply many times the nutritional content of the root. They are excellent sources of **vitamins** and **minerals**.

Turnips detoxify the body and alkalize the blood, promoting sweating, releasing mucous and improving the **appetite**. They are also generally beneficial in conditions such as indigestion, diabetes and jaundice. Turnip greens have traditionally been used in Asia in the treatment of lung congestions, bronchitis, asthma and sinus problems. Although raw turnips have a somewhat pungent smell, this is neutralized in cooking.

TYROSINE, L-TYROSINE

A non-essential amino acid, tyrosine has many vital effects in the body such as fighting depression, maintaining energy and controlling weight. Together with **iodine**, tyrosine produces thyroxine, the vital thyroid hormone that controls the rate of metabolism, weight, energy and growth. With **phenylalanine**, tyrosine produces norepinephrine (adrenalin) and **dopamine**, two important **neurotransmitters** – the chemicals that enable brain cells to communicate with each other. Norepinephrine is important in the control of stress, anxiety, fatigue and allergies, while dopamine controls motivation, movement and emotions. Tyrosine participates in the production of endorphins, the brain's natural pain relievers and mood elevators. Tyrosine is abundant in animal food and is also available as a nutritional supplement from health food stores.

Caution: Tyrosine should not be used by people with melanoma.

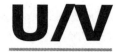

U/V

UMEBOSHI

Umeboshi is a Japanese salty-sour plum (ume). The **plums** are pickled with sea **salt** and sundried for three to four days in the hottest days of the summer, then pickled again with sisho leaves. Increasingly available in western health food shops, umeboshi is highly alkaline and antibiotic. It is revered in Japan as a digestive aid, blood purifier, general tonic and intestine regulator.

UVA URSI SEE BEARBERRY

VALERIAN (*VALERIANA OFFICINALIS*)

A wild herb with fragrant flowers, valerian is cultivated for its root and its essential oil. A tincture of the oil is well known as a strong sedative that counteracts anxiety, calms nervousness, and reduces heart palpitations, spasms and epileptic fits. Valerian is a wonderfully soothing herb which promotes sleep and is a good painkiller.

Traditionally used to prevent fainting, valerian can help in the treatment of digestive ulcers and reduce the urge to smoke. Available from health food stores, pharmacies and herbalists. Also widely incorporated in nutritional formulas.

Caution: Valerian should not be prepared as a **tea** unless prescribed by a doctor. Prolonged use of the herb can cause depression.

VALINE

An essential amino acid needed for the formation of **protein** in the body, valine has a stimulating effect. It is one of the three branched chain **amino acids** and, in combination with the other two, **leucine** and **isoleucine**, valine benefits muscles. It assists the repair of muscle tissue in cases of injury. Available from health food stores and in nutritional formulas.

VANADIUM

Vanadium has recently been discovered as an essential nutrient in human nutrition. Named after the Scandinavian goddess of beauty, vanadium is a trace element that appears to improve insulin action. Vanadium supplements (mostly as vanadyl sulphate) have improved **glucose** tolerance in animals, inhibited **cholesterol** and increased bone mineralization. As a result, vanadyl sulphate is now commonly used by diabetics. Vanadyl sulphate is found in many foods. Its best sources include **buckwheat, parsley, mushrooms**, black pepper, **dill** and **shellfish**. No deficiency symptoms of vanadium have been noted so far, but a daily intake of 10–60 mcg is considered normal. An upper limit was recently set at 1.8 mg a day.

VEGAN DIET

The vegan diet is a strict form of vegetarianism that promotes the use of fruits, vegetables and spring **water**, and excludes any animal foods, even those accepted by many **vegetarians**, such as dairy foods or **eggs**.

Vegan diets have proved beneficial in detoxifying the blood, preventing various diseases such as hypertension, high **cholesterol**, heart disease, cancer and osteoporosis, while curing inflammations and allergic conditions such as asthma and hay fever. Allergies and inflammations are known to arise from leukotrienes, metabolic derivatives of **arachidonic acid**. This is an essential fatty acid found exclusively in animal products. The elimination of animal products, as in the vegan diet, is thought to prevent the formation of leukotrienes and their related diseases. Obviously, a strict, long-term vegan diet is not suitable for everyone, and could create deficiencies in nutrients such as **vitamin B12, zinc** and **proteins**, leading to fatigue and anaemia. However, this effect can be avoided by the use of concentrated foods such as **brewer's yeast, bee pollen, spirulina, blue-green algae, chlorella**, or by taking supplements. Another way to avoid protein deficiency among vegans is to eat the correct plant protein combinations, for instance, by combining **grains** and **legumes** at the same meal and in the correct proportions to yield usable protein (see *Complete Nutrition*). Soya products such as **miso** and **tofu** are also very helpful for increasing protein intake. It should be remembered, however, that nutrient requirements vary from person to person, and that for many people strict dietary restrictions can cause nutrient shortages and deficiency symptoms unless supplements are used.

VEGETARIAN DIET

A vegetarian diet excludes the use of animal **meats**, but not necessarily the use of other animal products such as **eggs,** milk, yogurt and **cheese**. It depends on the individual interpretation of vegetarianism. However, all vegetarian diets are high in **fibre** and, usually, the **protein** problem is less acute than in the **vegan diet** since vegetarians use some animal protein, which supplies **vitamin B12**, and they also use high-protein soya products freely, such as **tofu** and **miso**. In general, vegetarian diets have been shown to be effective in lowering high **cholesterol** levels and hypertension, preventing atherosclerosis and heart disease, alleviating constipation and reducing the risk of colon cancer, breast cancer and kidney stones. A vegetarian diet can also help to prevent osteoporosis, since a high protein diet and sugar are known to increase excretion of **calcium** in the urine.

VERVAIN, VERBENA (*VERBENA OFFICINALIS*)

A herb that grows wild in meadows and roadside verges, it is also widely cultivated as a garden plant. It was traditionally regarded as a 'sacred' herb, and infusions of verbena leaves are used by both herbalists and homeopaths. Taken in a single dose, these infusions are diuretic, they loosen phlegm so that it can be coughed up, stimulate vomiting, promote perspiration, relieve indigestion, and can benefit ulcers and colitis. Vervain is also a sedative, relieving depression and anxiety, inducing sleep and alleviating certain types of migraine.

VINE LEAVES (*VITIS VINIFERA*)

Vine leaves are commonly used in Mediterranean cooking and contain important **bioflavonoids**, such as anthocyanidins which are potent **antioxidants**, and other flavonoids. These factors promote blood circulation, strengthen veins and capillaries, and help retain their flexibility. The leaves are also recommended in the treatment of varicose veins and haemorrhoids. Available from specialist ethnic grocers.

VITAMINS

Vitamins are micronutrients, a group of about 20 organic substances other than **proteins, carbohydrates, fats, minerals** or salts. Vitamins are extremely complex chemical substances. Being essential to human nutrition, they are found in minute amounts in foods. The first ones were discovered in 1911 by Dr Casimir Funk, but by now they have been isolated and synthesized.

Like their name implies, they contain a vital part, with an amine group attached. Vitamins do not contain **calories** and are not a source of energy, but they are vitally important as constituents of **enzymes**, the organic catalysts that release energy and sustain life. Vitamins are indispensable for normal metabolism, growth, well-being, body development and reproduction. Vitamins work together, enhancing each other's effects, and their shortage is known to cause **deficiency diseases**.

Vitamins are not formed in the body but must be supplied by plant or animal foods. The few exceptions include **vitamin A** which can be formed in the body from its precursor, **beta carotene; vitamin D** formed by the action of ultraviolet light on the skin; and **vitamin K** formed by intestinal bacteria. As a general rule, vitamins are unstable, easily destroyed by air, oxidation, heat, light, drugs and aging. Vitamins are broadly classified into water-soluble vitamins (such as the **B complex** and **C**) which are measured in milligrams, and fat-soluble vitamins (**A, D, E** and **K**) measured in international units (i.u.).

Although each one of us basically needs the same vitamins, we are all individuals biochemically. Personal requirements vary with metabolic rate, food intolerance, genetic makeup, lifestyle, sex, age and body size.

Requirements for vitamins A and C for example, can vary up to twentyfold between different people. Vitamins are seriously depleted in the body by smoking, **alcohol**, drugs, stress, the contraceptive pill, crash diets and by common diets rich in refined **carbohydrates** such as white sugar, polished **rice** and white flour, from which most vitamins have been removed during processing. Balancing diet shortages with vitamin supplements, above the Recommended Daily Allowances, is therefore highly recommended by nutritionists to prevent deficiency symptoms and sustain a feeling of well being. Megavitamin supplementation, that is, taking vitamins in extremely high doses for specific conditions, should be done only under the supervision of a qualified nutritionist.

VITAMIN A

Vitamin A is an **antioxidant**, fat-soluble vitamin that occurs in two forms. In animal foods such as **fish** oils and liver, it occurs as **retinol** which is readily used by the body or stored in the liver. In vegetable foods, it occurs as **beta carotene** and other **carotenoids** (provitamin A) which must first be converted in the body to retinol, before becoming usable as vitamin A.

Vitamin A is important for growth, development and fertility. It boosts the immune system and helps to fight colds, increasing resistance to infections of mucous tissue linings such as eyes, ears, throat, lungs and bladder. Together with beta carotene it improves vision, especially night vision, by forming a photosensitive pigment called visual purple. Vitamin A maintains a healthy-looking skin, preventing acne, dermatitis and skin cancer. High doses of retinol and beta carotene can also prevent cancer of the lungs, bladder and breasts. Deficiency symptoms include red itchy eyes, impaired vision, dry or rough skin and a predisposition to colds and infections.

Vitamin A is stored in the liver until needed and, in spite of its wide prevalence, deficiencies do occur. Most vulnerable are dieters, people on low fat regimes and **vegans**, since only a small part of the beta carotene is converted to retinol if the fat intake is low. Vitamin A supplements are therefore important in unbalanced diets. The Recommended Daily Allowance for adults is 5,000 i.u., and for children 3,000 i.u. Requirements increase during illness, but decrease when using oral **contraceptives**. Most nutritionists recommend a daily dose of 10,000 i.u. for adults. Excessive doses in the order of 50,000 i.u., taken regularly over periods of a few months, can produce toxic effects.

VITAMIN B COMPLEX

B complex is a group of water-soluble B vitamins that occur together in many vegetables and animal foods. Rich sources include liver, **brewer's yeast**, raw wheat germ and brown **rice**. Although certain functions of many B vitamins overlap, all have their own characteristics and they cannot replace one another. Moreover, they interact with each other in many bodily functions. They are vital for such activities as energy production, carbohydrate metabolism and proper nerve function. They have a wide range of effects, from alleviating stress to preventing atherosclerosis. Their deficiency symptoms include fatigue, nervousness, depression, anaemia, weak digestion, poor **appetite**, constipation, hair loss and high **cholesterol** levels.

B vitamins are depleted by refined sugar and flour, and by **alcohol** and, being water-soluble, the B vitamins in raw vegetables readily dissolve into the cooking water, enriching the soup or cooking liquid. It is important therefore to save the cooking water of vegetables or brown **rice** as this provides a rich source of B vitamins. When taking supplements of B vitamins, it is best to consume the whole B complex. Excessive supplementation of only one of the B vitamins disrupts the balance and can promote elimination of the others.

When a specific B vitamin is needed to treat a particular condition, say B6 for dieting, it is best to take an additional source of B complex in order to maintain a proper balance of the other B vitamins.

VITAMIN BI (*THIAMINE*)

This was the first B vitamin to be identified and, as it was discovered in **rice** husks, thiamine became commonly known as the cure for beri-beri, a fatal Asian disease caused by eating polished rice. It was realized that the symptoms of beri-beri, such as mental disturbances, muscle wasting, hypertension and heart attacks, could be cured simply by eating raw brown rice.

As a **coenzyme**, thiamine is essential for energy production, carbohydrate metabolism and nerve function. As an **antioxidant**, it can help to prevent arthritis and atherosclerosis caused by free radical damage. Together with **vitamin C** and **cysteine**, thiamine also helps to protect from the damage caused by smoking and smog.

Thiamine has been called the 'morale vitamin' due to its salutary effect on the nerves. It promotes a feeling of optimism, helps to overcome stress, depression, anxiety and poor memory, stabilizes **appetite** and maintains normal heart function; it is important to growth, lactation and fertility. Deficiency symptoms include fatigue, water retention, poor appetite, heart palpitations, low thyroid function, nervous exhaustion, irritability, fear, anxiety and confusion. Among the best natural sources of thiamine are **brewer's yeast, rice bran**, raw wheat germ, whole **grains, peanuts** and green and yellow vegetables. The vitamin is destroyed by **alcohol**, coffee, **tea** and raw **fish**.

The Recommended Daily Allowance is 1.4 mg for adults and 0.7 mg for children, but many people use supplements containing 50 mg to ensure a feeling of well-being Requirements increase during stress, lactation or illness.

VITAMIN B2 (*RIBOFLAVIN*)

First identified as the yellow-green pigment in **milk**, riboflavin is vital for metabolism and energy production. Together with **vitamin A**, it contributes to good vision and promotes growth and fertility. Large doses have been reported to prevent athlete's foot, improve eczemas and allergies, and counteract a sweet tooth.

Riboflavin is not destroyed by cooking, but it is sensitive to light – which is why milk, which is a good source of riboflavin, should not be kept in clear containers or exposed to strong sunlight.

Riboflavin deficiency symptoms include the cracking of the lips at the corner of the mouth, tongue inflammations, a sensation of sand in the eyes, cataracts, migraine, scaly skin on the face, dental problems, anaemia and heart disease. Among the best natural sources of the **vitamin** are milk, liver, **brewer's yeast**, dairy products, leafy green vegetables, **fish** and **eggs**. The Recommended Daily Allowance is 1.7 mg for adults and 1 mg for children, although most popular supplements contain 50 mg. Since riboflavin is excreted through the kidneys, excessive consumption or supplementation will result in yellowish-green urine, but this is perfectly normal.

VITAMIN B3 (*NIACIN*)

Also called nicotinic acid, niacin was discovered while searching for the cause of pellagra, a common endemic disease of the eighteenth century, which is characterized by the three Ds – dermatitis, dementia and diarrhoea. It is a water-soluble **vitamin** available in two forms, niacin and niacinamide.

Niacin assists metabolism, digestion and energy production, and improves blood circulation, preventing blood clots and heart attacks; it lowers high **cholesterol** levels effectively when taken in daily doses of 3 g or more and is vital to a healthy nervous system, alleviating nervousness, mental disorders and suicidal tendencies. It also enhances insulin secretion and has been reported to benefit new cases of diabetes. In higher doses of 50 mg, niacin releases histamine which produces a temporary hot skin flush for a few minutes. This reaction can be prevented by using niacinamide instead of niacin or by using 'flush free' niacin products. (Histamine is a chemical released during allergic reactions, but which is also vital to various functions of the body such as growth, wound healing and orgasm.)

Severe deficiencies of niacin can bring about the symptoms of pellagra, although nowadays this is somewhat rare. However, lower deficiencies are very common and symptoms can include fatigue, indigestion, bad breath, arthritis, headaches, high cholesterol levels and lost sense of humour.

Megadoses of a few grams of niacin a day have been used successfully to treat clinical depression and schizophrenia, and it is assumed that such illnesses are indicative of a much higher requirement for niacin. Niacin supplements have also been used to treat alcoholism and smoking.

Among the best natural sources of niacin are liver, **brewer's yeast, eggs, fish, rice bran, wheat bran, peanuts, sunflower seeds** and **wheat** germ. The Recommended Daily Allowance is 20 mg for adults and 13 mg for children. However, niacin supplementation of 50–100 mg a day can be safely used for greater benefits. Niacin and niacinamide supplements are available on their own or in B complex or multivitamin formulations. Niacin supplements are best taken with meals.

VITAMIN B5 SEE PANTOTHENIC ACID

VITAMIN B6 (*PYRIDOXINE*)

One of the busiest of the B vitamins, pyridoxine is an **antioxidant vitamin** and is involved with more than sixty **enzymes**, taking part in many varied metabolic functions. It promotes muscle energy by releasing stored sugar from the liver; it helps to metabolize **fats** and control obesity, lowers **cholesterol** and prevents atherosclerosis; it regulates the **sodium**–potassium balance, preventing water-retention; it maintains a correct acid–alkaline ratio and assists the functions of nerves. Pyridoxine also inhibits the release of histamine and is therefore beneficial to asthmatics and allergy sufferers, and it helps to synthesize **nucleic acids**, antibodies and red blood cells. In addition, it promotes healthy pregnancies, strengthens the immune system and assists blood formation. Pyridoxine supplements of 50 mg daily can effectively prevent morning sickness in pregnancy, and higher doses of 200 mg daily are reported to be effective in treating carpal tunnel syndrome, reducing the need for surgery. Pyridoxine is also involved in brain chemistry, promoting the production of **neurotransmitters** such as **serotonin**, and it has been found helpful for controlling occurrences of epileptic seizures. Together with **magnesium**, pyridoxine inhibits the formation of **oxalic acid** salts, such as calcium oxalate, thus helping to prevent kidney stones.

Pyridoxine is not stored in the body, and is depleted in **milk** by pasteurization, partially destroyed by cooking, and mostly removed from **grains** by refining. Alcohol and the contraceptive pill are among its greatest antagonists, and any woman on the pill should consider taking pyridoxine supplements. Deficiency symptoms include water retention, linear nail ridges, tongue inflammations, inability to tan, numbness of hands and feet, convulsions in children, depression, tremors, hypoglycaemia, diabetes, **appetite** loss, high **cholesterol** levels, kidney stones, osteoporosis, arthritis, allergies, asthma, anaemia and poor dream recollection.

Some of the best natural sources of pyrodoxine are **brewer's yeast**, liver and kidney, **sunflower seeds**, raw **wheat** germ, **walnuts, molasses, cabbage, milk** and **eggs**. The Recommended Daily Allowance for adults is

2.2 mg, and 1.7 mg for children. The normal nutritional supplementation range is between 50 and 100 mg daily. As it is a water-soluble vitamin, pyridoxine supplementation is best divided throughout the day and taken at intervals.

VITAMIN B12 (*COBALAMIN*)

Isolated from liver extract in 1948, vitamin B12 was identified as the food factor that prevents the fatal condition pernicious anaemia. The vitamin is water soluble and contains the mineral **cobalt**, hence its name. It comes in several forms, of which cyanocobalamin is the most common.

Although cobalamin is required in tiny amounts, measured in micrograms, it is essential for the functioning of all cells and is principally involved in energy metabolism, immune function and nerve function. Together with **folic acid**, the vitamin forms red blood cells to prevent anaemia, and promotes growth and **appetite** in children, increases energy, improves brain functions such as memory and learning ability, maintains a healthy nervous system, stabilizes menstruation and prevents post-natal depression. Vitamin B12 is used to treat a wide range of conditions, such as fatigue, depression, Alzheimer's disease, asthma, infertility, multiple sclerosis, noise-induced hearing loss and AIDS.

The absorption of B12 depends on a stomach secretion called the 'intrinsic factor'. Many people with reduced secretion suffer unknowingly from a deficiency of the vitamin, which can take years to manifest since B12 is stored in the liver – unlike the other water-soluble vitamins. B12 deficiency is thought to be especially common in the elderly, and affects primarily the brain and nervous system.

Apart from fatigue and depression, deficiency symptoms include a pins-and-needles sensation, impaired memory, red tongue, diarrhoea, shortness of breath, heart palpitation and apathy. More acute deficiencies include symptoms such as loss of co-ordination and senile dementia.

B12 is found in significant quantities only in animal products, and its richest sources are liver, kidneys, sardines, **eggs, fish** and cheese. In non-animal foods, B12 is found in fermented soya products (**miso, tofu, tempeh**), **algae** (**spirulina**, **chlorella**, **blue-green algae**) and **bee pollen. Vegans** and strict **vegetarians** are well advised to take B12 supplements to prevent deficiencies. The typical Recommended Daily Allowance is 2 mcg for adults and 1 mcg for children. Supplements are available in potencies of 60–2,000 mcg. Some people are not able to absorb B12 easily, and therefore need to take high supplementary dosages, either orally or by injection.

VITAMIN B15 SEE PANGAMIC ACID

VITAMIN C (*ASCORBIC ACID*)

Vitamin C is a water-soluble nutrient that was recognized as a cure for scurvy long before it was isolated in 1933. In recent years, it has received a great deal of public attention as a cure for the common cold. But vitamin C does much more than just prevent scurvy and colds. For example, as an **antioxidant**, it delays ageing and prevents age-related diseases from arthritis to Parkinson's disease; as an antihistamine, it alleviates allergies; and as an antipollutant, it eliminates toxins from the body.

However, the chief function of vitamin C is the production of collagen, the structural **protein** that holds our bodies together. As such, it hastens the healing of wounds, prevents bleeding gums and strengthens capillaries and blood vessels, preventing heart attacks and strokes.

Collagen is also the subcutaneous 'cement', and facial wrinkles can be a sign of a life-long deficiency in vitamin C. Vitamin C is also a powerful booster of the immune system and is well known for its ability to increase resistance to infection and disease by increasing the production of anti-bodies and interferon, which fight microbes and viruses. Scientific studies have confirmed that megadoses of vitamin C can reduce the risk of a wide range of cancers, and also inhibit tumour development and prolong the survival of cancer patients. In dosages of at least 1,000 mg a day, vitamin C helps to lower **cholesterol** by speeding its conversion to **bile**. Vitamin C also aids the absorption of **iron**, preventing anaemia and provides protection against the devastating effects of smoking and alcoholism.

Deficiency symptoms of vitamin C include susceptibility to colds, infections and allergies, easy bruising and the slow healing of wounds, inflamed gums and defective teeth, fatigue and anaemia, and nervousness, anxiety and depression. Among the best natural sources of the **vitamin** are fresh citrus fruits, **peppers, guavas, broccoli, Brussels sprouts, cabbage, papaya** and **kiwi**. The natural vitamin C in fruits and vegetables is highly perishable as the vitamin is unstable and disintegrates, not only in cooking, but also in peeled fruits and vegetables.

The Recommended Daily Allowances of vitamin C are 60 mg for adults and 45 mg for children. However, these are ridiculously low dosages and the main effect is to prevent scurvy. For optimal benefits, doses of a few grams a day are recommended. Vitamin C tablets that contain **bioflavonoids** are preferable.

VITAMIN D

Vitamin D is a fat-soluble vitamin, known as the 'sunshine vitamin' because the sun's ultraviolet rays convert subcutaneous **cholesterol** to vitamin D.

There are two major forms of vitamin D – D2 (ergocalciferol) and D3 (cholecalciferol). D2 is the form added to **milk**.

Vitamin D promotes the absorption of **calcium** and **phosphorus**, both vital for strong bones and teeth. It also assists the assimilation of **vitamin A** and maintains a healthy nervous sytem, normal heartbeat and efficient **blood clotting**. New research has shown that increasing the intake of vitamin D through exposure to sunlight or eating oily fish can help in the treatment of asthma, and provide protection against prostate cancer.

Vitamin D is mainly stored in the liver. Typical deficiency symptoms include porous bones (leading to rickets in children), tooth decay, fatigue and arthritis, and one report links myopia (short-sightedness) to vitamin D deficiency. The vitamin is scarce in vegetables and its best natural sources include **fish** liver oil, sardines, herring, **salmon**, tuna and fortified **milk**. The recommended daily allowance is 400 i.u. for adults and children.

Caution: Prolonged daily doses above 1,600 i.u. can lead to over-accumulation and toxicity symptoms such as diarrhoea, calcification of the arteries and kidney damage.

VITAMIN E

Vitamin E is a fat-soluble vitamin composed of a group of substances known as tocopherols, which are subdivided into alpha, beta, gamma, and so forth. Of these, alpha tocopherol is the most active. Vitamin E is available in both natural and synthetic forms, with the natural forms designated 'd' on supplement labels, as in d–alpha-tocopherol, and the synthetic forms designated 'dl', as in dl–alpha-tocopherol. The two forms are mirror images of one another, but only the natural 'd'-form is recognized by the body. 'Tocopherol' is derived from two Greek words meaning 'childbearing', since early studies of vitamin E involved fertility problems.

Vitamin E is a most important lipid **antioxidant**. It binds oxygen and protects the **fats** in our bodies from the damaging effects of uncontrolled oxidation, peroxides and free radicals. These peroxides attack body cells, immune cells and **cholesterol**, reducing resistance and causing the degenerative diseases of ageing, such as cancer, heart attacks, strokes, arthritis, senility and diabetes. By binding oxygen, vitamin E alleviates some of the primary causes of death and helps to extend life-span. Vitamin E improves cell respiration (a boon to joggers), promotes fertility and sexual potency, is very effective in preventing the hot flushes of menopause and miscarriages, and protects the body from common pollutants such as ozone, radiation and toxic elements. The vitamin is used in the treatment of many conditions, including atherosclerosis, angina, hypertension, cancer, haemolytic anaemia, allergies, cataracts, eczema, acne, premenstrual syndrome, skin ulcers, burns and digestive ulcers. A recent study has shown that a daily dose of 2,000 i.u. taken regularly can slow the deterioration resulting from Alzheimer's disease.

Vitamin E deficiency symptoms include fatigue and premature ageing, sterility and miscarriage, muscular dystrophy, haemolytic anaemia (which is not responsive to **iron** intake), circulatory disorders such as coronary thrombosis, varicose veins and thrombophlebitis, lameness due to poor circulation (claudication), kidney inflammation, degeneration of sex glands, and slow healing of wounds and burns. Among its best natural sources are raw **wheat** germ and **wheat germ oil**, vegetable oils, **soybeans**, whole **grains, eggs** and leafy green vegetables.

The Recommended Daily Allowance of vitamin E is 15 i.u. for adults and 10.5 i.u. for children. However, for optimal protection, much higher doses are recommended. Vitamin E is available in potencies between 100 i.u. and 1,000 i.u. on its own, and it is also included in nutritional formulas. The most popular daily supplement is 400 i.u.

VITAMIN K

A fat-soluble vitamin, vitamin K tends to be a neglected nutrient because it is rarely deficient. It is known for its role in producing blood-clotting factors, such as prothrombin and, in this way, it contributes to the prevention of internal haemorrhaging and reduces excessive menstrual flow. It is also used to prevent haemorrhagic diseases in **babies**. In addition, vitamin K has recently been found to promote the building of healthy bones and to prevent osteoporosis.

Vitamin K occurs in three forms: K1 (phylloquinone), the natural vitamin K from plants; K2 (menaquinone), derived from intestinal bacteria; and K3 (menadione), which is the synthetic version of vitamin K available for those who cannot absorb it from food. To ensure adequate absorption and production of vitamin K in the body, cultured **milk** products such as **yogurt** and buttermilk, as well as vegetable oils, should be included in the daily diet. Antibiotics and over-consumption of sugar and sweets inhibit vitamin K absorption.

Deficiency symptoms include delayed blood–clotting of wounds, haemorrhages such as nose bleeds, and a low level of blood platelets. Deficiencies of the vitamin are usually caused by a defect in metabolism, a malfunction of the liver, or by coeliac disease. Coeliac patients should emphasize vitamin K-rich foods in their diet and supplement with **vitamins** K, **A, D** and **E**, and also with **calcium** and the **B-complex** vitamins. The best natural sources of vitamin K include **kale**, green **tea, alfalfa, spinach, broccoli, lettuce, cabbage, watercress, yogurt**, egg yolk, **fish** liver oil and **soybean** oil. No official Recommended Daily Allowance has been established, but 300 mcg is generally considered adequate for an adult.

VITAMIN P SEE BIOFLAVONOIDS

VITEX, CHASTE TREE (*AGNUS CASTUS*)

Vitex is a shrub with finger–shaped leaves and violet flowers that grows on river banks in the Mediterranean region. A traditional European plant used already by ancient Greeks, its other name 'chaste tree' is derived from the belief that the ripe fruit of the plant would suppress the libido of women taking it.

Vitex was used for centuries in Europe to treat pre-menstrual syndrome (PMS) and the side effects of menopause. Although it does not contain hormones, it helps correct progestrone deficiencies and balance women's hormonal system. It stimulates the pituitary gland to increase production of luteinizing hormone. This in turn increases the level of progestrone during the second half of a woman's cycle, normalizing the oestrogen–progestrone ratio. Vitex also reduces high prolactin levels in the second half of the menstrual cycle which causes breast tenderness and pain. It is commonly used by European herbalists to treat female complaints such as irregular or excessive menstruation, amenorrhoea (lack of menstruation), infertility, menopausal hot flushes, fibroid tumors and cervical dysplasia (abnormal cell growth on the cervix as shown by Pap test). Vitex is now being rediscovered by women looking for a natural alternative to hormone replacement therapy (HRT).

Vitex is increasingly available in health food shops in liquid extracts which are taken in drops once daily. It is best used over a period of several months continuously. Once improvement has occurred, treatment should be continued for another month. Side effects are rare. Less than 2 per cent of the users reported a minor tummy upset and mild skin rash.

Caution: Vitex is not recommended during pregnancy or during HRT.

W

WAKAME (*Undaria pinnatifida*)

A popular dark-green Japanese seaweed, wakame grows
in wing-like fronds up to 50 cm (20 in) long in sea water.
Wakame is one of the **seaweeds** highest in **calcium** content
(more than 10 times the calcium of **milk**). It is also rich in
iron, thiamine and niacin. And as with all other seaweeds, it
contains small amounts of many **minerals** and trace elements
of the sea water. Wakame is widely available in health food
shops in its dried form.

Used in cooking, it can soften beans and the hard **fibres**
of foods cooked with it. Wakame is an indispensable part of
the Japanese diet and a basic component of **miso** soup. In
the Japanese tradition it is used to purify the mother's blood
after childbirth. A normal daily consumption of dry wakame,
before soaking with other foods, is 5–15 g.

WALNUTS (*Juglans nigra*)

One of the oldest food trees, walnuts have been used for
food and medicine throughout history. Two of its species,
the English walnut and the American black walnut, are the
most popular. Apart from the value of the tree as timber,
the walnuts are highly nutritious. They are rich in **protein**
and antioxidants, **vitamin E** and **minerals** such as **iron,
calcium, magnesium, manganese** and **phosphorus**.
Walnuts contain monounsaturated fats including **omega-3**

fatty acids and, uniquely, alpha-linolenic acid. Walnuts are known to help reduce the 'bad' LDL **cholesterol**. Walnuts also contain antioxidants, particularly ellagic acid, which help protect cells from free-radical damage.

WATER

The most vital nutrient in our bodies, water makes up two-thirds of the body's mass and is involved in nearly every bodily process. Good, pure water is not only enlivening but also nutritious. Pure water acts in the body as a solvent, lubricant and coolant. Recently, pure water was found to function as an electromagnetic enhancer.

As such, pure water reduces the risk of heart disease, helps release contaminants from fat cells assisting weight loss, and reduces water retention by dispersing salt, just like common diuretics. Although 'soft' water can be kinder to the skin when used externally, 'hard' water is nutritionally more beneficial to the body: it contains various **minerals**, especially **calcium** and **magnesium**, and is known to reduce the incidence of heart disease.

Unfortunately, contamination of tap water has become commonplace in recent years, due partly to the chemicals added at treatment plants and partly to contamination collected in the course of water distribution. Tap water is chlorinated and may cause allergies, diarrhoea or depression, as well as destroying friendly intestinal bacteria. It can also contain anti-corrosion chemicals added by some water boards, as well as environmental pollutants and industrial wastes. In addition, it may carry germs, algae, scale and rust particles which can contaminate the blood and lymph, overburdening the liver and kidneys with poisons, and lead to reduced energy and a lower resistance to disease. Since the purity and quality of water so greatly affects general health and well being, it is no wonder that there is a growing public demand for higher-quality water and that people are increasingly using bottled mineral waters, water filters and water purifiers.

As with any other nutrient, the body requires water in sufficient amounts. Insufficient water intake is known to promote constipation, an accumulation of toxins, kidney damage, fatigue, apathy and dehydration. **Meat**-based diets increase the need for water because they overload the body with urea and other toxic by-products of **protein** metabolism that need water for their dispersal and elimination. As a rule, **vegetarians** require less water than meat-eaters since many fruits and vegetables contain over 90 per cent water. Water is best drunk before or between meals. Water drunk right after meals can dilute digestive juices and is a common cause of heartburn.

Individual water requirements vary from person to person, and although thirst is considered the best indicator of need, it is often unreliable. On average, due to a gradual loss of the thirst sensation, we do not drink enough water. Yes, we drink a lot of sodas, **tea** and coffee, but all these cannot replace the body's demand for water. They only serve as vehicles to stimulating chemicals such as **caffeine, aspartame** and sugar. In his book, *Your Body's Many Cries for Water*, Dr F. Batmanghelidj presents his revolutionary concept that chronic dehydration of body cells can cause many diseases. He cites many varied conditions, like stomach ulcers, arthritis, headaches, hypertension, high **cholesterol**, diabetes and even obesity, all of which were successfully treated by drinking at least 2 l of water a day.

Caution: Do not self-treat the above conditions. Seek professional help.

WATERCRESS (*NASTURTIUM OFFICINALIS*)

A perennial herb of the **mustard** family, it grows naturally in running water, especially the beds of streams, but is grown commercially in watercress beds or is raised as a winter crop in greenhouses. Watercress is cultivated for its leaves, which are used mainly in salads and are rich in **vitamins** and **minerals**, especially **vitamins A** and **C, zinc** and **iron**. The plant is also rich in **potassium, calcium, phosphorus** and iron, with good quantities of **iodine, sodium** and **magnesium**.

Although the healing powers of watercress have long been known, recent scientific studies have shown that it can inhibit the growth of some cancerous tumours. New research has revealed that fresh watercress contains high levels of PEITC (phenethyl isothiocyanate), which neutralizes a dangerous carcinogen in tobacco called NNK and one study indicated that the consumption of 60 g of fresh watercress three times a day for three days will help to protect smokers from lung cancer. For more lasting protection, this process can be repeated once a month.

A **tea** prepared from the leaves can strengthen digestion, increase urination, and cleanse the respiratory system by releasing phlegm and mucus. Watercress is also recommended for the treatment of catarrh, anaemia, weak digestion and gout.

Caution: Excessive or prolonged use of watercress may cause kidney problems, and it should not be used in pregnancy. Since, nowadays, wild watercress grows mainly in polluted waters, it may contain various pollutants as well as the deadly liver fluke. Therefore, wild watercress is unsafe for gathering, and only watercress grown commercially in filtered, shallow, gravelled-bottom beds should be consumed.

WHEAT (*TRITICUM AESTIVUM*)

Traditionally termed 'the staff of life', whole wheat is a highly nutritious grain and includes several varieties, such as bulgur and durum. Wheat starch contains anywhere between 6 and 20 per cent **protein** made up of eight **amino acids**. Wheat germ is a rich source of **vitamin E, B vitamins** and **minerals** such as **zinc, iron, copper** and **iodine**. The **brain** is rich in **fibre** and the amino acid **lysine**. Wheat encourages growth and can be used in conditions such as nervousness, insomnia and irritability.

Being mildly astringent, wheat can be used for bed-wetting, diarrhoea and night sweats.

Sprouted wheat, particularly **wheat grass**, is an increasingly popular form of easily digested wheat.

Standard white flour is made from the inner starchy part of the grain, with all the germ and bran removed. This results in a loss of up to 80 per cent of the essential nutrients in wheat. In addition, white flour may be bleached with chlorine dioxide, which destroys all the vitamin E. 'Enriched' flours make up for only a few of the missing nutrients, usually vitamins B1, B2, B3 and iron.

Gluten, the elastic protein in wheat, is used as a popular source of vegetable protein in many dishes around the world. However, it can cause allergies and people with coeliac disease cannot digest it at all. The symptoms of coeliac disease, which is quite widespread, include diarrhoea, abdominal pain, flatulence, intestinal damage, weight loss and spasms. Coeliacs must not only avoid wheat, but all other gluten–containing cereals as well, and subsist on a gluten-free diet.

WHEAT GERM OIL

Produced from the life-giving part of the wheat kernel, wheat germ oil has been found to have many beneficial effects on the human body. It is the richest source of **vitamin E**, the great antioxidant and fertility vitamin. It is also the richest source of **octacosanol**, a type of waxy **alcohol**, the effects of which have a variety of effects on the body, including increased energy, endurance and strength, improved resistance to stress, alleviation of arthritis and improved heart function. In experiments done with the US Marines, wheat germ oil was found to relieve fatigue, dizziness, drowsiness and fear. In addition, animal studies have shown that wheat germ oil increases pregnancy rates and reduces miscarriages. Octacosanol has been found to have a remarkable therapeutic effect on muscular dystrophy and nerve-muscle disorders such as multiple sclerosis, epilepsy, cerebral palsy, encephalitis and myasthenia gravis. It has also been reported to regulate the **blood clotting** hormones, preventing blood clots and heart attacks.

The best wheat germ oil is cold pressed, fresh and packed in amber bottles. It is best kept in the refrigerator and taken in a dosage of a teaspoon on empty stomach, 1–3 times daily.

Caution: Wheat germ oil contains significant amounts of oestrogen, the female sex hormone, and large doses over a prolonged period can cause testicular degeneration and loss of sex drive in men. For higher levels of supplementation, octacosanol tablets are safer and more beneficial.

WHEAT GRASS (*AGROPYRON*)

Considered a 'living food', wheat grass is very rich in
vitamin E, chlorophyll and many nutrients. It cleanses the
blood, rejuvenates the body and increases resistance to disease.
It is a tonic and helps to treat conditions such as fatigue,
anaemia, toxaemia and cancerous growths.

Wheat grass juice is a powerful detoxifying agent. It helps
to increase the enzyme level in the body cells, aiding the
rejuvenation of the body and the digestion of
nutrients. Wheat grass juice is best taken fresh on an
empty stomach, starting off with 30 g a day, a daily dose that
can gradually be increased to 125 g. It is usually diluted with
carrot or **apple** juice to make it more palatable.

More common in the USA in larger health food stores
where it can be bought as freshly squeezed juice.

WHEY

Whey is the **water** separated from **milk** during cheese- making
after the milk has coagulated. It is considered highly nutritious
and is the richest source of **lactose** (milk sugar). It is often
added in dry form to processed foods, but is not suitable for
people with **lactose intolerance** or for those allergic to milk.

Whey has recently been found to contain certain
proteins that can speed up the healing of wounds and
ulcers. Initial studies were successfully conducted by
Australian scientists who plan to use these whey ingredients
in the form of dressings to accelerate wound repair. Other
studies suggest that whey proteins may have anti-cancer and
anti-microbial effects, as well as improving immune function.

Some products on the market already use whey. Estée

Lauder sells a moisturizer, called Nutritious, which uses whey protein to mimic a natural cellular messenger found in skin, which instructs it to produce more collagen. It is claimed that it makes the skin stronger and more supple.

WILD YAM SEE YAM

WINE

The oldest beverage known to man, written records on the dietary and therapeutic properties of wine date back 4,000 years. Most of today's wines come from a species of vine that originated in the Middle East, while many varieties were crossbred with species native to North America and Canada.

Drunk in moderation, wine appears to be more than just an alcoholic or romantic drink. Wine constituents have a relaxing effect and are known to promote the absorption of essential minerals like calcium, magnesium, phosphorus and zinc. Red wine has been found to increase blood levels of **HDL** ('good' cholesterol) while decreasing **LDL** ('bad' cholesterol), and recent scientific research has indicated that two glasses of red wine a day can help prevent blood clots, lower **cholesterol**, reduce the risk of heart attack and contribute to a longer life.

Red wine is brewed from whole **grapes**, with skin and seeds, unlike white wine, and contains important antioxidant polyphenolic flavonoids, such as **quercetin**, catechins and tannins. But the most exciting polyphenol found in wine is resveratrol, a natural plant antibiotic produced by plants to combat fungal and bacterial attacks. Red wine is particularly rich in resveratrol; one glass of red wine contains 650 mcg while a handful of peanuts contains only 75 mcg resveratrol. Recent clinical studies have shown that as a potent antioxidant, resveratrol not only helps protect the heart but also helps prevent cancer, reduce the risk of osteoporosis and alleviate depression.

Being a phytoestrogen, resveratrol was also found to act as a natural replacement for oestrogen and to improve menopausal symptoms like hot flushes and mood swings. And recent American research revealed that resveratrol can also help prevent herpes. The scientists found that dabbing the infectious sores with red wine can hamper their growth and can stop the sufferer passing it on. In general, higher concentrations of resveratrol are found in wines associated with cooler and more humid climates such as Burgundy, Bordeaux, Switzerland, Oregon and Canada, while wines from warmer and drier climates tend to have lower concentrations.

Red wine is known to cause headaches or nasal congestions in some people and, although a controversial issue, it is suspected that these are allergic reactions to sulphites which are added to the wine to inhibit oxidation and microbial growth. Although most wine makers add sulphites, an increasing number are going 'organic', producing wine with no additives. (See also GRAPES.)

WITCH HAZEL (*HAMAMELIS VIRGINIANA*)

A deciduous tree, native to North America, it was traditionally endowed with magical properties, hence its name. It is now grown in many other temperate regions of the world, including the British Isles.

The leaves of the witch hazel have an astringent, tonic and

sedative effect. A decoction can be used for diarrhoea. Extracts of witch hazel, which are available from most herbalist, should be used only externally. As a skin lotion, the extract can be applied to bruises, insect bites and
minor sunburn. A poultice is said to help in the treatment of haemorrhoids. The decoction can also be used as a mouth-wash and as a vaginal douche for vaginitis. Available from health food stores and herbalists.

WORMWOOD (*ARTEMISIA ABSINTHIUM*)

A silky perennial herb prevalent in arid roadside verges in Europe and North America, the leaves and flower tops of wormwood are used for several conditions. The leaves contain herbal bitters and santonin, which is effective against intestinal worms, and are used to prepare a bitter oil and also infusions. Wormwood is antiseptic and carminative, and can be used to stimulate the **appetite** and to treat indigestion. Wormwood oil is a cardiac stimulant and improves blood circulation.

Caution: Pure wormwood oil is poisonous and should be used only in correct dosages as indicated by a herbalist. Available from larger health food stores and herbalists.

Y

YAM, WILD YAM (*DIOSCOREA VILLOSA*)

Wild yam is a perennial vine with a tuberous rootstock that is
native to North America. Its roots yields an alkaloid
which is a muscle relaxant, and it was used to treat
abdominal cramps and bilious colics during the American
Civil War. It can also be used to regularize menstruation
and relieve menstrual cramps. One particular species of
wild yam, *D. vitata*, has been found to contain up to 40
per cent diosgenin, a glycoside that can easily be converted
to the hormone progesterone. (This hormone was
previously produced from horse's urine.) In a study carried
out over a four-year period, wild yam was found to be
effective as an oral **contraceptive**, but without the side
effects of the pill.

YARROW (*ACHILLEA MILLEFOLIUM*)

A herb that commonly grows wild along roadside verges,
yarrow contains an essential oil and two acids, which
together produce an astringent infusion that is aromatic
and has a bitter taste. Traditionally, yarrow **tea** was used
to induce sweating during a cold, and it is still
recommended by herbalists for this purpose. An infusion
of the plant can be used to alleviate digestive upsets, and
arrest internal bleeding and heavy menstrual flow.

Externally, it can be used as a soothing application for

wounds, sore haemorrhoids, and also as a mouthwash in cases of gum inflammation and as a hair tonic. It is widely available from herbalists.

Caution: Yarrow can cause dermatitis in some people.

YEAST SEE BREWER'S YEAST

YOGURT

Increasingly publicized as a health food, yogurt has been used for centuries by many of the long-living ethnic societies. Now rediscovered as a **probiotic** food, yogurt is simply **milk** that has been fermented by several strains of bacteria, such as *Lactobacillus acidophilus* and *Bifidobacteria bifidum*. The bacteria curdle the **milk** by converting the milk sugar to lactic acid. One of the main nutritional benefits of yogurt is to reinforce the intestines with additional 'friendly' bacteria, promoting the growth of intestinal flora. The bacteria of the intestinal flora aid digestion and absorption of food, produce **B vitamins**, prevent the growth of pathogenic bacteria (such as candida) which cause diseases, and inhibit internal decay; they also promote a healthy intestinal acidity. In this respect, yogurt is especially beneficial to people on **antibiotics**, and for those who have a sweet tooth or who drink chlorinated **water**, all of which deplete friendly bacteria. Yogurt also helps to synthesize **vitamin K**, preventing internal haemorrhages, and it lowers **cholesterol** levels and reduces the risk of cancer, especially colon cancer.

However, apart from these benefits, yogurt is also a highly nutritious food. It is a good source of quality

protein, vitamins and **minerals**: it contains **vitamins A, B complex, E and D**, is an excellent source of easily absorbed **calcium, potassium** and **phosphorus**, and contains only a moderate amount of **sodium**. Yogurt is also easily digested – in fact, most of its **protein** is digested within an hour. It is also a highly valuable food for the treatment of gastro-enteritis, colitis, constipation, bilious disorders, flatulence, bad breath, high **cholesterol**, migraine and nervous fatigue. In addition, yogurt can often be taken by people who cannot use other forms of milk due to **lactose intolerance**.

YOHIMBE (*PAUSINYSTALIA JOHIMBE*)

In recent years, yohimbe capsules have swept health food stores in the USA as a potent aphrodisiac. The bark of the yohimbe plant, which is a native of South America, contains yohimbine, and this was approved by the US FDA for the treatment of erectile dysfunction. Although yohimbine can increase sex drive, its primary action is to increase blood flow to the erectile tissue. It has no effect, however, on testosterone levels. When used on its own, yohimbe can help about a third of cases. However, its side effects, which include depression, anxiety, hallucinations, headaches, hypertension, dizziness and skin flushing, make it difficult to use. Both yohimbe and yohimbine are therefore best used under medical supervision.

Z

ZINC

An essential trace element, zinc is found in every cell of
the body and performs numerous useful functions. It is
a component of some 200 **enzymes** and is involved in
more enzymatic reactions than any other mineral. It is
a constituent of **insulin, growth hormones** and sex
hormones, and is richly contained in human sperm. It takes
part in carbohydrate metabolism, the breakdown of **alcohol**
and the synthesis of **nucleic acids**. Together with **vitamins
A, B6** and **B12**, zinc is necessary for proper growth. It also
aids the excretion of toxic **cadmium** found in cigarette
smoke (which causes hypertension), and neutralizes the bad
effects of excess **copper** (a cause of arthritis). Zinc is crucial
to the maturation of the sex glands and for their function,
particularly the prostate. It prevents enlargement of the
prostate, which can block urine flow and is a source of distress
for many men over 45.

Together with **vitamin B6**, zinc inhibits histamine
production and is therefore helpful in treating allergies. It
soothes nerves and depression and is used in the treatment
of Alzheimer's disease and some types of schizophrenia.
Zinc can also speed up the healing of wounds and is used
to cure ulcers resulting from cortisone treatment. Due to its
presence in insulin, zinc increases the insulin effect and is
therefore helpful in the treatment of diabetes. It has also
been found to boost natural immunity against disease, and
is well-known for its ability to promote skin health and

alleviate psoriasis. For this reason, it is sometimes used as an ingredient in skin creams.

The symptoms of zinc deficiency are many and varied. They include swollen prostate, sterility and impotence, and delayed sexual maturation in children, stunted growth, menstrual irregularities, susceptibility to infections and poor wound healing, joint pains, atherosclerosis and poor circulation, slow learning and mental retardation, loss of sense of taste and smell, allergies, acne, stretch marks in pregnant women, white spots in the nails, offensive perspiration, and susceptibility to diabetes.

Zinc is depleted by **alcohol** and smoking, and profuse sweating can cause a loss of up to 3 mg a day. Among the best natural sources of the mineral are raw **oysters**, clams, **meat, fish**, raw wheat germ, **brewer's yeast, mushrooms, pumpkin** seeds, egg yolks and **legumes**. The Recommended Daily Allowance is 15 mg for adults and 10 mg for children. Requirements increase during pregnancy or lactation. Zinc supplements in strengths of up to 40 mg are available in health food stores.

HELPFUL ADDRESSES FOR GENERAL HERBAL ADVICE

UK

The British Herbal Medicine Association (BHMA), Sun House,
Church Street, Stroud, Gloucestershire GL5 1JL

The National Institute of Medical Herbalists, 9 Palace Gate,
Exeter, Devon EX1 1JA

The Herb Society, 77 Great Peter Street, London SW1,
www.herbsociety.co.uk

General Council and Register of Consultant Herbalists, Grosvenor
House, 40 Sca Way, Middleton-on-Sea, West Sussex PO22 7SA

USA

The American Botanical Council, P.O. Box 201660, Austin, Texas 78720

The Herb Research Foundation, 1007 Pearl Street, Suite 200, Boulder,
Colorado 80302

American Herb Association, P.O.B. 353, Rescue, CA 95672 California
School of Herbal Studies, P.O.B. 39, Forestville, CA 95436

Australia

National Herbalist Association of Australia, 27 Leith Street, Coorparoo,
Queensland 4151

HERBAL SUPPLIERS

UK

Potters Herbal Suppliers, Leyland Mill Lane, Wigan, Lancashire WN1 2SB
Tel: 0942 34761

Culpepper Ltd, www.culpepper.co.uk

Neal's Yard Remedies, 15 Neal's Yard, Covent Garden, London
WC2H 9DP Tel: 020 7379 7222

A. Nelson & Co. Ltd, www.nelsonshomeopathy.co.uk

USA

Nature's Herbs, 113 North Industrial Park Drive, Orem, Utah 84057
Tel: 801 225 4443

Nature's Way, 1375 N. Mountain Springs Parkway, Springville, Utah
84663 Tel: 801 489 1500

Eclectic Institute, 11231 S.E. Market Street, Portland, Oregon 97216
Tel: 800 332 4372

Wakunaga, 23501 Madero, Mission Viejo, California 92691 Tel: 800 544
5800

Acta Health Products, 1979 East Locust Street, Pasadena, California
91107

Four Seasons Herb Company, 17 Buccaneer Street, Marinal Del Rey,
California 90292 (specializes in oriental herbs)

Bio-Botanica, Inc., 75 Commerce Drive, Hauppauge, New York 11788
Tel: 516 231 5522

Earthrise Company, P.O. Box 1196, San Rafael, California 94915
Tel: 415 485 0521

Threshold, 23 Janesway, Scotts Valley, California 95066 Tel: 408 438 1144

Excel, 3280 West Hacienda, Las Vegas, Nevada 89041 Tel: 702 795 7464

Yerba Prima, P.O. Box 5009, Berkeley, California 94705 Tel: 415 632
7477

Canada

Trophic Canada Ltd, 260 Okanagan Avenue East, Penticton, BC V2A357
Tel: 604 492 8820

Flora Distributors Ltd, 7400 Fraser Park Drive, Burnaby, BC VSJ5B9
Tel: 604 438 1133

Swiss Herbal Remedies, 181 Don Park Road, Markham, Ontario
L3RIC2 Tel: 416 475 6345

Quest, 1781 West 75th Avenue, Vancouver, BC V6P6P2 Tel: 604 261 0611

The Herb Works, PO Box 450, Fergus, Ontario N1M1N8 Tel: 519 824
4280

Vita Health, 150 Beghin Avenue, Winnipeg, MBR1J3W2 Tel: 204 661
8386

Bio-Force, 4001 Cote Verth, Montreal, PQ H4R1R5 Tel: 514 335 9393

INDEX

322

336